RENAL D

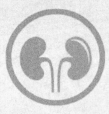

COOKBOOK

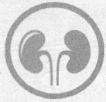

FOR BEGINNERS

2024

Delicious & Easy-to-Make Recipes Low in Sodium, Potassium & Phosphorus to Manage Kidney Disease. Eat Healthfully & Tasty by Swapping Your Daily Routine with a 6-Week Meal Plan

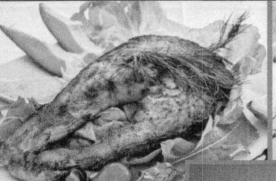

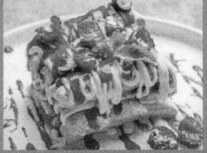

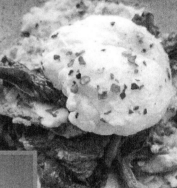

6 - WEEK
MEAL PLAN

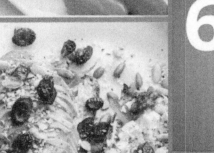

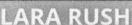

LARA RUSH

1500
DAY RECIPE

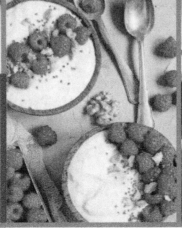

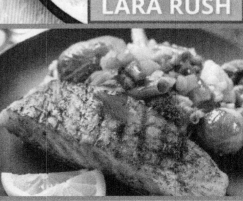

Renal Diet
Cookbook

3 IN 1

Delicious & Easy-to-Make Recipes Low in Sodium, Potassium & Phosphorus to Manage Kidney Disease. Eat Healthfully & Tasty By Swapping Your Daily Routine with a 6-Week Meal Plan!

Lara Rush

Table Of Contents

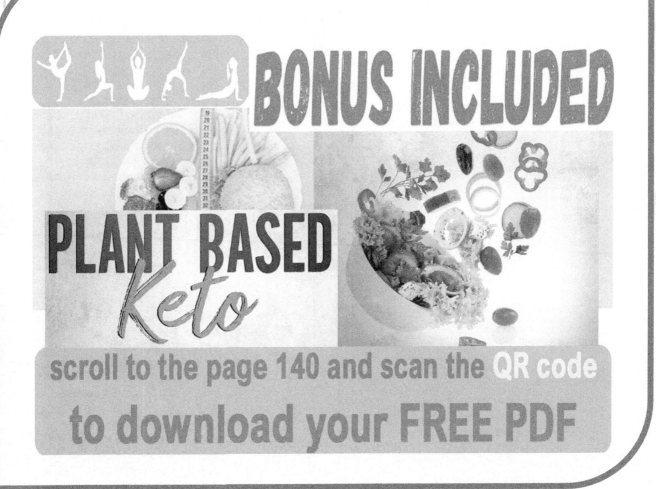

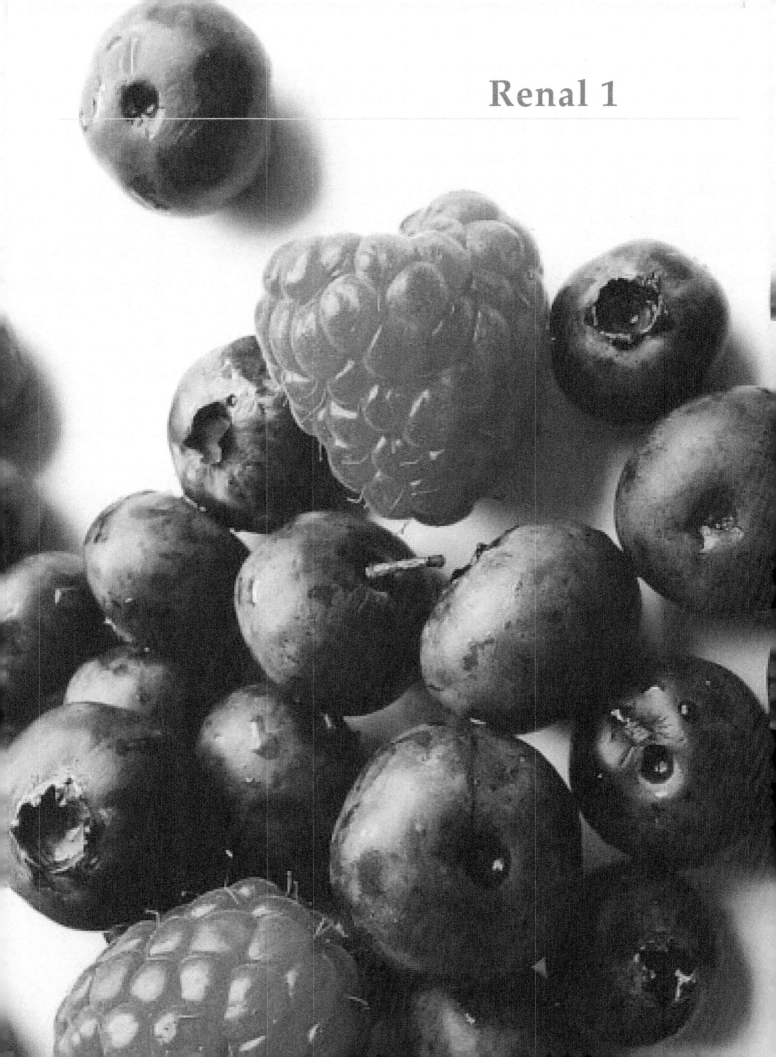

Renal 1

Introduction

At any stage of our existence, food is essential for the good health of the body, as well as in the prevention of diseases. In the case of kidney disease, maintaining a balanced eating plan is essential to reduce the risks of these diseases: kidney failure, kidney stones, among others.

The proper functioning of the kidneys will depend largely on the food we eat. A consistent diet must provide the body with the substances necessary for health, and these ingredients are classified into macronutrients and micronutrients.

Macronutrients are responsible for providing energy. In this group, we find carbohydrates, proteins, and fats. On the other hand, micronutrients are foods rich in vitamins, minerals, fiber, and even water.

The System Needs Balance

In this case, for the urinary system and the rest of the body to function optimally, it is necessary to maintain a balance of these food groups: macronutrients and micronutrients. That balance is known as homeostasis. Therefore, it is necessary to adapt new eating habits taking into account the capabilities of the kidneys.

When we eat foods high in fat without any type of control, this surplus will accumulate in adipocytes, unlike micronutrients. However, the deficiency or excess of minerals and vitamins also leads the body to suffer from other pathologies.

The blood must contain stable concentrations of minerals, vitamins, proteins, and water for the optimal functioning of the organism, and the kidneys are in charge of this balance in the blood.

Kidney Diseases

In those with problems of urinary system diseases, it is necessary for them to know the classification of foods, vegetables, and fruits. If food is not suitable for these individuals, certain substances will accumulate in the blood because they cannot be expelled through the urine.

For example, a diet high in protein can produce hyperfiltration that could further deteriorate the kidney situation, requiring greater effort. A healthy eating plan must be followed to reduce cardiovascular risk factors and diabetes, obesity, high cholesterol, also responsible for aggravating kidney disease, even requiring dialysis or a kidney transplant.

Likewise, it should be noted that a diet plan for a kidney patient will depend on the stage of the disease (predialysis, dialysis, kidney transplantation), and the diet must be modified according to the clinical conditions of the patient.

At the beginning of kidney disease, once the filtering capacity of the kidneys to eliminate toxins is diminished, feeding care must be further increased. For example, dialysis patients need to consume more protein.

Dialysis is responsible for filtering the blood in a similar way, but not as effective as the kidneys would. With dialysis, fluid can build up in the body, which means a decrease in fluid consumption to prevent any inflammation in the extremities, stomach, and even under the eyes.

Likewise, it can increase blood sugar levels, since the liquid used for dialysis contains high levels of glucose, requiring the patient, in addition to medical treatment for kidney failure, other diabetes medications.

In this book, we have compiled special recipes for people with kidney problems. This eating plan is designed to consume up to approximately 2,000 calories a day, combining the appropriate servings of cereals, dairy, protein foods, vegetables, and legumes.

Likewise, you should increase your fluid intake and reduce salt and sodium. As for the consumption of protein, this should be in small amounts. Dairy should not exceed ½ cup of milk or yogurt or a slice of cheese.

RENAL DISEASE

The kidneys perform a great function in our body. They are in charge of filtering and eliminating all the waste and excess fluid that are within your body. They also maintain a healthy balance of water, salts, and minerals (sodium, calcium, phosphorus, and potassium) in the blood.

That is why the correct functioning of these organs allows us to enjoy good health and stability in our system. But the failure of one or both can have serious health consequences, which, if not treated in time, can become chronic or even lead to death. That is why below we will explain in more detail what kidney disease is, all its implications, causes, and how to lead a healthy and full life if you suffer from this disease.

What Is Kidney Disease?

Over the years, our entire body ages, which also includes our internal organs. As time passes, their work capacity and efficiency decrease, which is a natural process that occurs in all animals. But this aging process is accelerated when the intake of food, liquids, or substances is incorrect, that is, when the body is not provided with the necessary nutrients for its proper functioning. Processed food, alcohol, tobacco, foods high in sugar and/or fat, and drugs, among other things, cause premature aging of our body, and in many cases, cause serious diseases. And our kidneys are not exempt from these phenomena.

The daily intake of alcohol, not ingesting the necessary amount of water per day (or exceeding its intake), or having a high intake of foods with a high percentage of proteins make our kidneys have to "work excessively," and this reduces their useful life. If these bad habits are maintained, it is very likely that the kidneys become ill and, at a point, they will no longer be able to adequately filter all the toxins and other waste substances found in the blood. These wastes will remain in the blood and the blood supply will take care of carrying them throughout your body, damaging other organs, and may irreversibly affect the brain and heart.

There are different types of kidney diseases and stages (which we will explain in the next section) but they all have symptoms in common, and among the most common are:

- Blood pressure increases due to fluid overload and the production of vasoactive hormones created by the kidney through the renin-angiotensin system, which increases the risk of developing hypertension and heart failure.
- Urea builds up, causing azotemia and ultimately uremia (symptoms ranging from lethargy to pericarditis and encephalopathy). Due to its high systemic concentration, urea is excreted in eccrine sweat in high concentrations and crystallizes on the skin as the sweat evaporates ("uremic frost").
- Potassium builds up in the blood (hyperkalemia with a variety of symptoms including malaise and life-threatening cardiac arrhythmias). Hyperkalemia usually does not develop until the glomerular filtration rate falls below 20 to 25 mL/min/1.73 m2, at which point the kidneys have a decreased ability to excrete potassium. Hyperkalemia in CKD can be exacerbated by acidemia (leading to extracellular potassium shift) and a lack of insulin.
- Symptoms of fluid overload can range from mild edema to life-threatening pulmonary edema.
- Hyperphosphatemia is the result of poor phosphate elimination in the kidney. Hyperphosphatemia contributes to increased cardiovascular risk by causing vascular calcification. Circulating fibroblast growth factor 23 (FGF-23) levels progressively increase as the renal capacity for phosphate excretion decreases, which may contribute to left ventricular hypertrophy and increased mortality in people with CKD.
- Hypocalcemia is the result of 1,25 dihydroxyvitamin D3 deficiency (caused by high FGF-23 and reduced kidney mass) and resistance to the action of parathyroid hormone. Osteocytes are responsible for the increased production of FGF-23, which is a potent inhibitor of the enzyme 1-alpha-hydroxylase (responsible for the conversion of 25-hydroxycholecalciferol to 1.25-dihydroxyvitamin D3). Later, this progresses to secondary hyperparathyroidism, renal osteodystrophy, and vascular calcification that further impair cardiac function. An extreme consequence is the appearance of a rare condition called calciphylaxis.
- Changes in bone and mineral metabolism that can cause 1) abnormal metabolism of calcium, phosphorus (phosphate), parathyroid hormone, or vitamin D; 2) abnormalities in bone turnover, mineralization, volume, linear growth or strength (renal osteodystrophy); and 3) vascular or other soft tissue calcification. The bone and mineral disorders of CKD have been associated with unfavorable outcomes.
- Metabolic acidosis may be due to a decreased ability to generate enough ammonia from the proximal tubule cells. Acidemia affects enzyme function and increases the excitability of cardiac and neuronal membranes by promoting hyperkalemia.
- Anemia is common and is especially prevalent in those who require hemodialysis. It is multifactorial but includes increased inflammation, reduced erythropoietin, and hyperuricemia leading to bone marrow suppression. Hypoproliferative anemia occurs due to inadequate production of erythropoietin by the kidneys.
- In later stages, cachexia can develop, leading to involuntary weight loss, muscle atrophy, weakness, and anorexia.
- Sexual dysfunction is very common in both men and women with CKD. Most men have a reduced sex drive, difficulty getting an erection and reaching orgasm, and problems worsen with age. Most women have problems with sexual arousal and painful menstruation and problems having and enjoying sex are common.

- People with CKD are more likely than the general population to develop atherosclerosis with subsequent cardiovascular disease, an effect that may be mediated at least in part by uremic toxins. People with CKD and cardiovascular disease have a worse prognosis than those with only cardiovascular disease.

Stages of Kidney Disease

Chronic kidney disease (CKD) is a type of kidney disease in which there is a gradual loss of kidney function over a period of months to years. Initially, there are usually no symptoms. Later on, symptoms may include leg swelling, feeling tired, vomiting, loss of appetite, and confusion. Complications include an increased risk of heart disease, high blood pressure, bone disease, and anemia.

The causes of chronic kidney disease include diabetes, high blood pressure, glomerulonephritis, and polycystic kidney disease. Risk factors include a family history of chronic kidney disease. Diagnosis is made by blood tests to measure the estimated glomerular filtration rate (eGFR) and a urinalysis to measure albumin. An ultrasound or kidney biopsy may be done to determine the underlying cause. Several severity-based staging systems are used.

Detection of people at risk is recommended. Initial treatments may include medications to lower blood pressure, blood sugar, and cholesterol. Angiotensin-converting enzyme (ACE) inhibitors or angiotensin II receptor blockers (ARBs) are generally first-line agents for blood pressure control, as they slow the progression of kidney disease and the risk of heart disease. Loop diuretics can be used to control edema and, if necessary, to further lower blood pressure. NSAIDs should be avoided. Other recommended measures include staying active and certain dietary changes, such as a low-salt diet and the right amount of protein. Treatments for anemia and bone disease may also be required. Severe disease requires hemodialysis, peritoneal dialysis, or a kidney transplant to survive.

Chronic kidney disease has 5 stages:

- **Stage 1:** Kidney damage is small and kidney function is normal. The patient may have high blood pressure, leg swelling, urinary tract infections, or abnormal urinalysis. The kidneys work at 90% of their capacity or more.
- **Stage 2:** Mild loss of kidney function. The patient may have high blood pressure, leg swelling, urinary tract infections, or abnormal urinalysis. The kidneys work between 60% and 89% of their capacity.
- **Stage 3:** This stage is divided into two sub-stages: 3a and 3b. In the first, the patient presents mild to moderate loss of renal function, the kidneys function between 45% and 59% of their capacity. And in the second stage, there is a moderate to a severe loss of kidney function, where the kidneys are working between 30% and 44% of their capacity. In both stages, the patient may present with low blood counts, malnutrition, bone pain, unusual pain, numbness or tingling, decreased mental alertness, or a feeling of discomfort.
- **Stage 4:** Here, the patient has a severe loss of kidney function, with their kidneys functioning between 15% and 29% of their capacity. Symptoms are anemia, decreased appetite, bone disease, or abnormal blood levels of phosphorus, calcium, or vitamin D.
- **Stage 5:** Here, the patient already has an end-stage renal disease (ESRD), where there is a need for dialysis or transplantation since their kidneys function below 15% of their capacity. Symptoms include uremia, fatigue, shortness of breath, nausea, vomiting, abnormal thyroid levels, swelling of the hands/legs/eyes/lower back, or pain in the lower back.

In summary, the most serious kidney diseases develop slowly, and in their most advanced stages, it is when the most noticeable symptoms and the urgent need for an operation appear. To detect this type of disease, laboratory studies using blood and urine samples are necessary, but if you have several of these symptoms together, do not hesitate and go to your family doctor or the nearest medical center.

How to Naturally Prevent the Need for Dialysis

Dialysis is the process of removing excess water, solutes, and toxins from the blood in people whose kidneys can no longer perform these functions naturally. This is known as kidney replacement therapy. The first successful dialysis was done in 1943. Dialysis may need to be started when there is a sudden and rapid loss of kidney function, known as acute kidney injury (formerly called acute kidney failure), or when a gradual decline in function kidney becomes chronic kidney disease and reaches stage 5. Stage 5 chronic kidney failure is reached when the glomerular filtration rate is 10–15% of normal, creatinine clearance is less than 10 ml per minute, and there is uremia. Dialysis is used as a temporary measure either in acute kidney injury or in those awaiting kidney transplantation and as a permanent measure in those for whom a transplant is not indicated or possible.

Dialysis is based on the principles of solute diffusion and fluid ultrafiltration through a semi-permeable membrane. Diffusion is a property of substances in water; substances in water tend to move from an area of high concentration to an area of low concentration. Blood flows through one side of a semi-permeable membrane and a dialysate, or special dialysis fluid flows through the opposite side. A semipermeable membrane is a thin layer of material that contains holes of various sizes or pores. Smaller solutes and fluid pass through the membrane, but the membrane blocks the passage of larger substances (for example, red blood cells and large proteins). This replicates the filtering process that takes place in the kidneys when blood enters the kidneys and the larger substances are separated from the smaller ones in the glomerulus.

The two main types of dialysis, hemodialysis and peritoneal dialysis, remove waste and excess water from the blood in different ways. Hemodialysis removes waste and water by circulating blood outside the body through an external filter, called a dialyzer, which contains a semi-permeable membrane. Blood flows in one direction and dialysate flows in the opposite. The countercurrent flow of blood and dialysate maximizes the solute concentration gradient between blood and dialysate, helping to remove more urea and creatinine from the blood. The concentrations of solutes normally found in the urine (for example, potassium, phosphorus, and urea) are undesirably high in the blood, but low or absent in the dialysis solution, and constant replacement of dialysate ensures that the concentration of solutes unwanted remains low on this side of the membrane. The dialysis solution has levels of minerals such as potassium and calcium that are similar to their natural concentration in healthy blood. For another solute, bicarbonate, the level of the dialysis solution is set at a slightly higher level than in normal blood, to stimulate the diffusion of bicarbonate in the blood, to act as a pH buffer to neutralize metabolic acidosis which is often present in these patients. The levels of dialysate components are usually prescribed by a nephrologist according to the needs of each patient.

In peritoneal dialysis, waste and water are removed from the blood within the body using the peritoneum as a natural semi-permeable membrane. Waste and excess water move from the blood, through the peritoneal membrane, and into a special dialysis solution, called dialysate, in the abdominal cavity.

To reach this critical point in where your kidneys need external ways to clean your blood, I recommend you follow the following steps:

- Avoid all foods that are high in salt.
- Avoid tobacco.
- Check your blood pressure regularly.
- Exercise regularly.
- Avoid foods with high percentages of fat, especially processed foods.
- Avoid consuming alcohol.
- Drink the amount of water necessary according to your age and body mass.

Following these simple steps will not only prevent your kidneys from deteriorating further, but your overall health will improve dramatically.

ESTABLISHING NEW HABITS

Set a Smart Goal

These types of radical changes are difficult to implement, especially after hearing the news that you have kidney failure. Therefore, far from being discouraged or setting unrealistic goals, the best option is to set clear, achievable goals with a deadline. In this way, you will stay focused on this new goal and it will become more bearable than if you set a totally unrealistic goal that involves making big changes and sacrifices in a short time.

Also, remember that all of this is a process that is not always linear and that there will be times when you may be tempted to eat unhealthy foods, but remember that your health is at stake.

For Kidney Failure: What Suggestions to Follow?

Cholesterol is a fat-like substance found in the blood. Your body needs cholesterol in certain amounts. Your body can make cholesterol and also get it from eating meats and other food products of animal origin. Too much cholesterol in the blood is bad. Too much cholesterol can build up in your blood vessels. This buildup can narrow your vessels and cause a blockage, preventing blood from reaching certain parts of your body. When this happens in the heart vessels, it is called coronary heart disease, and it can cause a heart attack. In people with chronic kidney disease (CKD), heart disease is very common and is the number one cause of death in this group. It is suggested that people with CKD have a cholesterol test every year. It is possible that your doctor wants to do them more often if something has changed with your health.

Low-density lipoprotein (LDL) cholesterol, also known as bad cholesterol, is the main cholesterol test used to detect heart disease. Other lab tests generally include:

- High-density lipoprotein (HDL) cholesterol, also known as good cholesterol.
- Triglycerides.
- Total cholesterol.

Since the results of these tests are affected by food, it is recommended that you do not eat for 9 to 12 hours before the laboratory tests are performed. Cholesterol lab values are different for adults and children. The lab ranges shown below are for adults and should not be used for children. People with good LDL cholesterol, high HDL cholesterol, and normal triglycerides are less likely to have heart disease. In addition to high levels of LDL cholesterol, the risk of heart disease increases with the following risk factors:

- Smoking cigarettes.
- Obesity.
- High blood glucose.
- Low HDL cholesterol.
- Age (men > 45 years; women > 55 years).
- High blood pressure or medications to control high blood pressure.
- Diabetes.
- Family history of early heart disease.
- Other diseases that affect the blood vessels.

People with CKD may have some additional risk factors that lead to heart disease:

- High intake of calcium from diet or medications.
- High levels of phosphorus in the blood.
- High levels of parathyroid hormone.
- High levels of homocysteine.
- Swelling of the whole body.

People who are physically inactive or who eat foods high in saturated fat and cholesterol are also more likely to develop heart disease. You are also recommended to:

- Increase physical activity to 30 minutes every day at a moderate level. This will help:
  - Raise HDL cholesterol.
  - Lower LDL cholesterol in some people.
  - Low blood pressure.
  - Improve blood glucose.
  - Improve heart function.
- Maintain a healthy weight.
- Talk to your doctor and dietitian.
- Do not smoke.
- Choose foods low in saturated fat and cholesterol.
- Decrease the use of trans fatty acids as they can raise LDL cholesterol.

- Use plant stanols and sterols found in specially formulated regular or "light" spreads like margarine. Increase soluble fiber. Fruits, vegetables, and grains are good sources of fiber.
- Talk to your dietitian to help you safely and gradually increase the fiber in your diet.
- Control high blood pressure and diabetes. Treatment for these conditions may include medications, changes in diet, and increased physical activity. Your healthcare professional can help you with lifestyle changes to better treat these conditions.
- Choose lean meats, poultry, and fish. Loin and round cuts of meat tend to be leaner than rib cuts and organ meats.
- Trim all visible fat from meat and remove the skin from poultry.
- Steam, broil, or bake meats, poultry, and fish. Place the food on a wire rack to allow the fat to drain off the food. Do not fry food.
- Choose fresh fruits and vegetables. Steam, boil, bake, or microwave vegetables. Do not fry food.
- Use nonstick skillets or vegetable sprays for sautéing.
- Use herbs and spices to flavor foods instead of sauces, butter, or margarine.
- Try wine, lemon juice, or flavored vinegar for low-fat, low-calorie flavor.
- Use gelatin, jam, honey, or syrup instead of butter or margarine on toast, waffles, pancakes, or muffins.
- Use fat-free or reduced-fat versions of high-fat foods. For example, use fat-free sour cream instead of regular sour cream or use skim or 1% milk in allowable amounts.
- Limit hydrogenated and partially hydrogenated fats. These can be found in some kinds of margarine, peanut butter, packaged baked goods and snacks, and fried foods. Try baked cookies instead of fried cookies. Buy grilled or baked foods when you eat out.
- Use 2 grams of plant stanols or sterols per day. These are sold as specially formulated margarine-like spreads. Your dietitian can help you find these products.
- Limit products made with coconut, palm kernel, palm oil, lard, shortening, bacon fat, and cocoa butter.
- Use canola or olive oil instead of lard, butter, or other oils when cooking. These monounsaturated fats will not lower your HDL level.
- Try ice cream or sorbet instead of ice cream.
- Read food labels. Don't be fooled by foods that are "cholesterol-free" but contain large amounts of saturated fat that your body will convert to cholesterol.

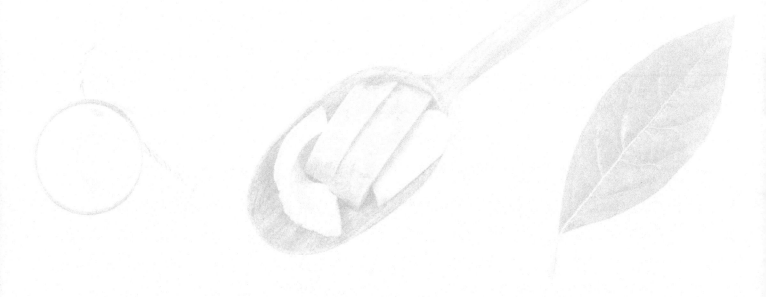

DIET

Control Your Diet

You should have a kidney-friendly eating plan when you have chronic kidney disease (CKD). Watching what you eat and drink will help you stay healthier. The information in this section is for people who have kidney disease but are not on dialysis. This information should be used as a basic guide. We are all different and we all have different nutritional needs. Talk to a kidney dietitian (a diet and nutrition expert for people with kidney disease) to find an eating plan that works for you. Ask your doctor to help you find a dietitian. Medicare and many private insurance policies will help pay for dietitian appointments.

What you eat and drink affects your health. Maintaining a healthy weight and eating a balanced diet low in salt and fat can help you control your blood pressure. If you have diabetes, you can help control your blood sugar by choosing what you eat and drink carefully. Controlling high blood pressure and diabetes can help prevent kidney disease from getting worse.

A kidney-friendly diet can also help protect your kidneys from further damage. A kidney-healthy diet limits certain foods to prevent minerals from those foods from building up in your body. With all eating plans, including the kidney-friendly diet, you need to keep track of the number of certain nutrients you eat, such as:

- Calories
- Protein
- Fats
- Carbohydrates

To ensure that you are getting the correct amounts of these nutrients, you must eat and drink the correct portion sizes. All the information you need to track your intake is on the "Nutrition Facts" label.

Use the Nutrition Facts section on food labels to learn more about the foods you eat. Nutrition facts will tell you how much protein, carbohydrates, fat, and sodium are in each serving. This can help you choose foods that are high in the nutrients you need and low in the nutrients you need to limit.

When looking at the nutrition information, there are a few key areas that will give you the information you need:

- Your body gets energy from the calories you eat and drink. Calories come from the proteins, carbohydrates, and fats in your diet. The number of calories you need depends on your age, gender, body size, and activity level. You may also need to adjust the number of calories you eat based on your weight goals. Some people will need to limit the calories they eat. Others may need to consume more calories. Your doctor or dietitian can help you figure out how many calories to eat each day. Work with your dietitian to come up with an eating plan that helps you get the right amount of calories and stay connected for support.

- Protein is one of the building blocks of your body. Your body needs protein to grow, heal, and stay healthy. Too little protein can weaken your skin, hair, and nails. But having too much protein can also be a problem. To stay healthy and help you feel better, you may need to adjust the amount of protein you eat. How much protein you should eat depends on your body size, activity level, and health problems. Some doctors recommend that people with kidney disease limit protein or change their protein source. This is because a diet that is very high in protein can make the kidneys work harder and cause more damage. Ask your doctor or dietitian how much protein to eat and what are the best sources of protein for you. Use the list below to find out which foods are low or high in protein. Keep in mind that just because a food is low in protein, it is not healthy to eat unlimited amounts.

- Carbohydrates are the easiest type of energy for your body to use. Healthy sources of carbohydrates include fruits and vegetables. Unhealthy carbohydrate sources include sugar, honey, hard candy, soda, and other sugary drinks. Some carbohydrates are high in potassium and phosphorus, which you may need to limit depending on the stage of kidney disease. We will talk about this in more detail later. You may also need to watch your carbohydrates carefully if you have diabetes. Your dietitian can help you learn more about the carbohydrates in your meal plan and how they affect your blood sugar level.

- You need some fat in your eating plan to stay healthy. Fat gives you energy and helps you use some of the vitamins in your food. But too much fat can lead to weight gain and heart disease. Try to limit the fats in your meal plan and choose healthier fats when you can. Unsaturated fats can help lower cholesterol. If you need to gain weight, try eating more unsaturated fats. If you need to lose weight, limit unsaturated fats in your meal plan. As always, moderation is the key. Too much "good" fat can also cause problems. Saturated fats, also known as "bad" fats, can raise your cholesterol level and increase your risk of heart disease. Limit them in your meal plan. Instead, choose healthier unsaturated fats. Trimming the fat from meat and removing the skin from chicken or turkey can also help limit saturated fat. You should also avoid trans fats. This type of fat increases "bad" cholesterol (LDL) and lowers "good" cholesterol (HDL). When this happens, you are more likely to have heart disease, which can cause kidney damage.

Sodium (salt) is a mineral found in almost all foods. Too much sodium can make you thirsty, which can cause bloating and raise your blood pressure. This can further damage your kidneys and make your heart work harder. One of the best things you can do to stay healthy is to limit the amount of sodium you eat. To limit sodium in your meal plan:

- Do not add salt to your food when you cook or eat. Try cooking with fresh herbs, lemon juice, or other spices without salt.

- Choose fresh or frozen vegetables over canned vegetables. If using canned vegetables, drain and rinse to remove excess salt before cooking or eating.
- Avoid processed meats like ham, bacon, hot dogs, and cold cuts.
- Eat fresh fruits and vegetables instead of crackers or other salty snacks.
- Avoid canned soups and frozen dinners that are high in sodium.
- Avoid pickled foods, such as olives and pickles.
- Limit high-sodium condiments like soy sauce, BBQ sauce, and ketchup.

Be careful with salt substitutes and "low sodium" foods. Many salt substitutes are high in potassium. Too much potassium can be dangerous if you have kidney disease. Work with your dietitian to find foods that are low in sodium and potassium.

Choosing healthy foods is a great start, but eating too much of anything, even healthy foods can be a problem. The other part of a healthy diet is portion control or watching how much you eat. To help control your portions:

- Check a food's Nutrition Facts label for the serving size and amount of each nutrient in a serving. Many packages have more than one serving. For example, a 20-ounce bottle of soda is actually 2 ½ servings. Many fresh foods, such as fruits and vegetables, do not come with Nutrition Facts labels. Ask your dietitian for a list of nutrition facts for fresh foods and tips on how to measure the correct portions.
- Eat slowly and stop eating when you are no longer hungry. It takes about 20 minutes for your stomach to tell your brain that it is full. If you eat too fast, you may eat more than you need.
- Avoid eating while doing something else, like watching TV or driving. When you are distracted, you may not realize how much you have eaten.
- Do not eat directly from the package the food came in. Instead, take out a serving of food and put the bag or box away.

Good portion control is an important part of any meal plan. It's even more important in a kidney-friendly eating plan, because you may need to limit the number of certain things you eat and drink.

Tips for Minerals and Vitamins

When your kidneys don't work as well as they should, waste and fluids build up in your body. Over time, waste and excess fluid can cause heart, bone, and health problems. A kidney-friendly eating plan limits the number of certain minerals and fluids you eat and drink. This can help prevent debris and fluid from building up and causing problems. How strict your meal plan should depend on the stage of your kidney disease. In the early stages of kidney disease, you may have little or no limit to what you eat and drink. As your kidney disease worsens, your doctor may recommend that you limit:

- Potassium.
- Phosphorus.
- Fluids.

Potassium is a mineral found in almost all foods. Your body needs some potassium for your muscles to work, but too much potassium can be dangerous. When your kidneys are not working well, your potassium level may be too high or too low. Having too much or too little potassium can cause muscle cramps, problems with the way your heart beats, and muscle weakness. If you have kidney disease, you may need to limit the amount of potassium you eat. Ask your doctor or dietitian if you need to limit potassium. Use the list below to find out which foods are low or high in potassium. Your dietitian can also help you learn how to safely eat small amounts of your favorite high-potassium foods. Eat the following low potassium foods:

- Blueberries
- White rice
- Red meat
- Onions
- Cauliflowers
- Strawberries
- Lettuce
- Apples
- Peppers
- Pineapple
- Chicken

And try to avoid the following high-potassium foods:

- Artichokes
- Integral rice
- Bananas
- Winter squash
- Spinach
- Beans
- Melons
- Oranges
- Avocados
- Raisins

- Potatoes
- Bran and granola products
- Tomatoes

Phosphorus is a mineral found in almost all foods. It works with calcium and vitamin D to keep your bones healthy. Healthy kidneys keep the right amount of phosphorus in your body. When your kidneys are not working well, phosphorus can build up in your blood. Too much phosphorus in the blood can cause weak bones that break easily.

Many people with kidney disease need to limit phosphorus. Ask your dietitian if you need to limit phosphorus. Depending on the stage of your kidney disease, your doctor may also prescribe a medicine called a phosphate binder. This helps prevent phosphorus from building up in the blood. A phosphate binder can be helpful, but you will still need to keep an eye on the amount of phosphorus you are consuming. Ask your doctor if a phosphate binder is right for you. Use the lists below to get some ideas on how to make healthy choices if you need to limit phosphorus.

You need water to live, but when you have kidney disease, you may not need as much. This is because damaged kidneys do not remove excess fluid as they should. Too much fluid in your body can be dangerous. It can cause high blood pressure, bloating, and heart failure. Excess fluid can also collect around the lungs and make it difficult to breathe. Depending on the stage of your kidney disease and your treatment, your doctor may tell you to limit fluids. If your doctor tells you this, you will need to reduce the amount you drink. You may also need to cut down on some foods that contain a lot of water. Soups or foods that melt, such as ice, ice cream, and gelatin, have a lot of water. Many fruits and vegetables are also high in water content. Ask your doctor or dietitian if you need to limit fluids. If you need to limit fluids, measure your fluids and drink from small glasses to help you keep track of how much you have drunk. Limit sodium to help reduce thirst. Sometimes, you may still feel thirsty.

Following a kidney-friendly eating plan can make it difficult for you to get all the vitamins and minerals you need. To help you get the right amounts of vitamins and minerals, your dietitian may suggest a special supplement for people with kidney disease. Your doctor or dietitian may also suggest a special type of vitamin D, folic acid, or iron pill, to help prevent some common side effects of kidney disease, such as bone disease and anemia. Regular multivitamins may not be healthy for you if you have kidney disease. They may have too many vitamins and too few. Your doctor or dietitian can help you find the vitamins that are right for you.

Important! Tell your doctor and dietitian about any vitamins, supplements, or over-the-counter medications you are taking. Some can cause more damage to your kidneys or cause other health problems.

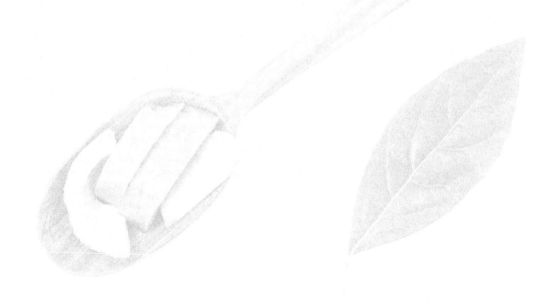

PHYSICAL EXERCISE

The Benefits of Physical Activity for Your Health and Your Kidneys

Exercise is important for people with chronic kidney disease (CKD) because when your kidney function has decreased, it can affect your muscles and bones. You can:

- Feel tired/without energy.
- Feel weak.
- Have joint pain.
- Have trouble breathing.

With regular exercise, you can control many of the health problems seen with kidney disease.

Some of the benefits of regular exercise are:

- More energy.
- Greater strength.
- Lower risk of falls.
- Able to walk further.
- Improvement of blood sugar levels and blood pressure.
- Improvements in restless leg symptoms.
- Weight loss.

What Kind of Exercise Should I Do?

Aerobic exercise is the best type of exercise for your heart because it helps strengthen your heart and lungs. Include activities like biking, walking, and swimming. Canada's physical activity guidelines encourage adults to get 30 to 60 minutes of aerobic activity 5–7 times a week, but every movement counts!

Resistance training is a type of exercise that strengthens your muscles. Repeat movements with weights or resistance tubes. Resistance training is especially important for people with CKD, as it helps prevent muscle weakness and joint pain.

Flexibility exercises prevent stiffness and increase mobility. They must be done in conjunction with resistance training. You hold the muscles in different positions for 30 seconds.

Balance exercises help reduce the risk of falls. Hold simple standing poses for 5 to 25 seconds to increase leg stability.

How Do I Start?

It is important to speak with your doctor before beginning an exercise program. That way, your doctor can guide you in choosing exercises that will help you, not hurt you. Be patient; it takes time to see results!

There are other benefits that you may not be able to see, so keep going! You will get the most benefits if you exercise regularly.

Common Questions

I Have Spoken With My Doctor. Now, What Do I Need to Know Before Starting?

Always start each exercise session slowly for at least 5 minutes before increasing your pace. Starting at a slower pace prepares the heart and lungs for the exercise session. Also, always slow down for a few minutes before stopping your exercise session. This will prevent you from feeling lightheaded or dizzy after exercising.

How Should I Progress in My Exercise?

You should always progress your exercise slowly. Start with 5–10 minutes of activity and add 1–2 minutes to your time each exercise session. Do this until you are exercising for as long as you want.

Is It Normal to Feel Pain After My Exercise Sessions?

It is normal to feel some muscle pain after exercise. Sometimes, new exercises use muscles that we haven't used in a long time, so they hurt. Remember that you should not feel pain during exercise. If you do, stop the exercise and talk to your doctor.

Other Benefits of Physical Activity

Being inactive increases the risk of developing long-term health problems, such as heart disease, stroke, diabetes, cancer, dementia, depression; the list seems to get longer all the time. In fact, being inactive is quite risky behavior!

Exercise Is Medicine!

In addition to helping prevent health problems, exercise is now used as part of the treatment of many of the diseases mentioned above. But what about kidney disease? Research shows that proper exercise is beneficial for kidney patients, but many kidney patients do not have the opportunity or believe that they cannot exercise. But most can exercise, and exercise can have benefits for adults of all ages. It will help you feel better, stronger, and in more control of your health. You just have to adapt the exercise to you and your circumstances. Whether you want to return to work, perform daily household activities, or manage your own health care, exercise will help.

Exercise Helps Protect the Heart

Having kidney disease also increases your chances of developing heart disease. Taking care of your heart is particularly important, for example, by quitting smoking and keeping your blood pressure and cholesterol levels under control. Plus, regular exercise really helps protect your heart and keep it in good shape by reducing your blood pressure, controlling cholesterol, preventing diabetes, and improving the condition of blood vessels.

Exercise Keeps Your Muscles Strong

People with kidney disease often find that they feel weaker and more tired than before and that their muscles tend to shrink and wear out. This happens to everyone if they don't use their muscles and keep them strong, but it can be worse if their kidneys are not working properly due to the extra toxins in the blood. Muscles are really important to everyone, not just weightlifters and gym bunnies, but anyone who just wants to be able to move around, climb stairs, or get up from a chair. Muscles are also important for overall health because they control how the body uses blood sugar and fats. Having good muscles and using them regularly really helps prevent diabetes and keep your heart healthy.

Exercise Helps You Live a Better Life

Physical activity can help you keep doing the things you enjoy that are important to you, whether it's playing a round of golf, taking your grandchildren to the park, going to the shops on a Saturday afternoon, or being able to walk up the stairs and take care of yourself in your own home. If you are not active, your fitness will decline and there will come a time when you will no longer be able to do these things. Everyone has the ability to improve their physical condition and become stronger, no matter where they start from. In fact, the least active people tend to see the greatest improvements when they exercise. So, have you decided to prepare yourself for a better and healthier life? What should you do? And where and how can you do it? This book answers some of the questions you may have and will help you establish an exercise program that is tailored to your needs.

Getting Started With Physical Activity and Other Tips

Talk to the People Involved in Your Care

They can tell you which exercise is best for you because they know your condition and treatment and what you can and cannot do. Your caregivers will probably be very happy if you ask them about exercise. Consult your doctor or healthcare professional, especially if you have:

- Kidney disease or more advanced kidney failure.
- Other health problems in addition to kidney disease, for example, heart or liver conditions, or difficulties with blood pressure control.
- Problems that affect your mobility or balance.
- Diabetes—Exercise can help diabetes, but you should ask about how to control your blood sugar levels, and please, take care of your feet.

Plan Your Exercise Program

To improve your health and fitness, it is important to gradually increase the amount of activity you do as your fitness improves and activities become easier. It is important to plan:

- What kind of exercises are you going to do.
- Approximately, the total time you spend exercising and the time or number of times you will do each exercise.
- How hard you work. For example, how fast will you walk or what weight will you lift.
- How often do you exercise.

Type of Exercise

A good exercise program consists of three different types of exercise: cardiovascular/aerobic (for the heart, lungs, and blood vessels, and also known as aerobic), endurance (for the muscles), and stretching (for flexibility). Each of these has different health benefits and you should try to do a few of each type.

Heating and Cooling

All exercise should always begin with a gentle warm-up with some light cardiovascular activity (for example, light walking) for about 10 minutes. Then you can work harder for a while before slowing down again to cool down and relax towards the end. Finish with some stretching.

Cardiovascular Exercise

This is a continuous activity like walking or biking, using large muscles, especially the legs. It benefits your whole body and makes you feel good. Think about what kinds of things you enjoy. Try to exercise for 30 minutes straight. However, if you can't handle this, to begin with, it doesn't matter, just do what you can and try increasing the time a little bit each week. You can do two 15-minute sessions or three 10-minute sessions in one day instead of one 30-minute session if that works better for you. Most people like to walk. This is an ideal exercise and a good way to start. Others may want to do something else, like ride a bike, swim, dance, or use gym equipment. It's up to you! You can combine different types of exercise on different days.

Endurance Exercise

This is where you move some kind of resistance (like your body weight or a dumbbell) in a way strong enough that you can only do it a few times. Resistance exercise is used to strengthen the muscles, but it will also benefit the whole body. Kidney patients often suffer from muscle weakness, and resistance exercise can help with this. Building stronger muscles will help you do other forms of exercise more easily and will also help you with your daily activities.

If you go to the gym, you can use the machines and equipment there; ask the staff to show you how. But you can also do resistance training at home, using simple things like cans of beans! Just follow a simple guide. Lift weights slowly, with very controlled movements, and continue until your muscles tire; this will tell them they need to get stronger. Choose a weight that you can lift 10 to 12 times before you have to rest; you may need lighter or heavier weights for different exercises. Keep breathing normally, don't hold your breath, and avoid lifting weights above your head. Focus on the large muscles in your lower body (legs), as these are the ones that will help you the most in your daily activities.

Elongation

Stretching is something that almost all patients can do. It is important to keep your joints running smoothly and preserve your full range of motion. Having a flexible body will help you with all your daily activities, as well as make exercise easier. We have included some stretching exercises for you in this guide. Perform each stretch to the point where you can feel the tension, but without causing pain. Hold the position for 20–30 seconds. In the last 10 seconds, you can try increasing the stretch a little more. Make sure to keep your body in good posture while stretching (look at photos to see how this should be done). Breathe normally and do not hold your breath.

How Long to Exercise

For your cardiovascular exercise, aim for, at least, 30 minutes a day for 3–4 days a week. It should gradually reach this level; don't try to do 30 minutes all at once to start. It is just as effective to do 2 or 3 shorter sessions at different times of the day (but each session should be at least 10 minutes to count towards the total). However, there is nothing magical in 30 minutes. If you feel like walking for 45 to 60 minutes, go for it. Just be sure to follow the tips listed under *How Hard to Exercise?* and *What Are the Signs That I Should Stop Exercising?* in this guide.

How Often to Exercise

For cardiovascular exercise, 3 days a week is the minimum requirement to achieve the benefits. Ideally, these would be non-consecutive days—for example, Monday, Wednesday, and Friday, but you can do more if you want. For resistance exercises, you should do them 2–3 times a week. You may find it easier to do your cardio and resistance exercises on different days. You can do your stretching exercises every day as you shouldn't find them strenuous. It's a good idea to include them in the warm-up and cool-down portions of your other exercise sessions.

How Hard to Exercise?

When you exercise, you need to make sure that you are doing enough work to benefit your health and increase your ability to do the things you want to do in life. But don't do so much that it hurts or makes you feel bad. This can be difficult without knowing your own exercise capacity. Generally, the following tips are helpful:

- For cardiovascular exercise, your breathing should not be so difficult that you cannot speak to someone who is exercising with you. (Try to find an exercise partner, like a family member or friend.) For resistance and stretching, you must breathe normally.
- After exercise, you shouldn't feel so much muscle pain that it prevents you from exercising for the next session.
- The most important thing is to start slowly and progress gradually allowing your body to adapt to the increased level of activity.

When counseling patients on how hard they should exercise, we use a scale based on exercise intensity, called the "Borg 15-Point Rate of Perceived Exertion Scale," or RPE. The RPE scale ranges from 6 to 20. At point 6, you would be sitting idle. At point 20, you would have exercised so much that you were exhausted and couldn't do more. You should aim for a consistent exercise rate, between 12 and 14. As you exercise, rate yourself against the RPE chart and think about how hard you are trying. How much effort are you putting in, how is your breathing, and how do you feel? If you rate an 11 on the scale, fairly light, try to exercise more to get to 12, 13, or 14. If you rate a 17, you will probably need to exert yourself less on your exercise. As your fitness increases, you should find that you can do more work on the "moderately difficult" scale of 12 to 14.

Don't be nervous or think it will be too difficult. Many people with kidney failure say they are too tired to exercise. They think that, if they exercise, they will be even more tired. The fact is that even a little exercise, 15–20 minutes a day, will actually help you feel less tired. Start slow and do what you can; you are not aiming to become a marathon runner. As long as you continue to do it regularly (at least 3–4 times a week), you will gradually get stronger and be able to do more and more.

Build Endurance—Cardiovascular Exercises

You don't need expensive equipment to do resistance exercises. You can use things that are in your house. If you use milk bottles you can vary their weight by filling them with more or less liquid. Food cans are also suitable for weighing. Follow the instructions below and start with a fairly light weight to begin to feel the movement, then increase the weight to make it more challenging. Maintaining proper technique is important when performing resistance exercises. Use the strength of the part of the body that each exercise is intended to work (described in the next few pages) and avoid rocking your body or bending or arching your back to lift a heavier weight. If you find yourself balancing the weight while lifting or bending and arching your back to lift a weight, stop and choose a lighter weight to avoid injury. This will also help you work the target muscle.

Some Exercises for You

BICEP CURL

Muscles that are worked: The front part of the arms.
Main muscle worked: Biceps.
1. Sit or stand upright holding your weight at your side.
2. Keep your elbows at your sides, bend your arms at the elbows, and bring your hands toward your shoulder.
3. Repeat as many times as you think you can.

PUSH UP ON THE WALL

Muscles worked: Back of arms and chest.
Main muscle worked: Triceps and pectorals.
1. Stand straight in front of a wall.
2. Place both hands on the wall at shoulder height.

3. Lean forward by bending your elbows until your nose almost touches the wall.
4. Push away from the wall until it is upright.
5. Repeat as many times as you think you can.

CHAIR SQUAT

Muscles that are worked: The butt and the front of the thighs.

Main muscle worked: Gluteus maximus and quadriceps.

1. Stand in front of a sturdy chair, reach back, and place your hand on your arms for balance.
2. Keep your feet shoulder-width apart and go to sit, but do not sit fully in the chair.
3. Hold this position for a few seconds and push back with your legs to stand up.
4. Repeat as many times as you think you can.

CLIMB STEP

Muscles worked: The front of the thighs.

Main muscle worked: Quadriceps.

1. Stand straight in front of a small step.
2. Hold something close to you if you wish, or place both hands on your hips.
3. Go up the step with your right foot and then your left.
4. Back up with the right and then with the left.
5. Repeat as many times as you think you can.

BACK LEG SWING

Muscles worked: The back of the legs and the back.

Main muscle worked: Hamstrings, gluteus maximus, erector spinae.

1. Stand straight in front of a chair and hold the back for support.
2. Keeping your back straight, bring one leg back, pointing your toes.
3. Slowly return your foot to the floor.
4. It is important not to arch your back.
5. Repeat as many times as you think you can, then switch and do the same with the opposite leg.

LOWER LEG EXTENSION

Muscles worked: The front of the thighs.

Main muscle worked: Quadriceps.

1. Sit upright with both feet flat on the floor.
2. Hold the seat for support.
3. Lift one leg off the ground and keep it straight.
4. Bend your knee and slowly lower your foot to the ground.
5. Repeat as many times as you think you can, then switch and do the same with the opposite leg.

HEEL LIFT

Muscles worked: Lower legs (calves).

Main muscle worked: Gastrocnemius.

1. Stand in front of a chair and hold onto the back for support.
2. With both feet, raise your heels and stand on the balls of your feet.
3. Slowly get back on your feet.
4. If you find this easy, put your hands on your hips.
5. Repeat as many times as you think you can.

THRUST

Muscles worked: The butt and the inside of the thighs.

Main muscle worked: Gluteus maximus and quadriceps.

1. Find something to hold onto, for example, a broom.
2. Step your left foot forward with the heel of your back foot slightly off the ground.
3. Keeping your back straight, bend your front knee keeping it on your foot.
4. Hold for a few seconds and push up.
5. Repeat as many times as you think you can, then repeat using the other leg.

NECK STRETCH

Muscle worked: The neck.

Main muscles: Sternocleidomastoid, trapezius, splenium.

1. Sit or stand straight facing forward.
2. Slowly, lower your right ear to your right shoulder.
3. Raise your head again and lower your left ear to your left shoulder.
4. Repeat a few times until your neck muscles feel looser.

HEAD TURN

Muscle worked: The neck.

Main muscles: Sternocleid-mastoid, splenium.

1. Slowly, turn your head to the right looking over your right shoulder.
2. Slowly turn your head back.

3. Then turn your head to the left to look over your left shoulder.
4. Slowly return your head to the center.
5. Repeat a few times until your neck muscles feel looser.

. SHRUG

Muscles worked: Shoulders, chest, and upper back.
Main muscles: Trapezius, pectorals.

1. Sit or stand upright.
2. Shrug your shoulders to your ears, hold and repeat.

ARM STRETCH AND WRIST ROTATION

Muscles worked: Arms, wrists, and shoulders.
Main muscles: Wrist flexors and extensors.

1. Sit or stand upright.
2. Start with your arms straight at your sides.
3. Raise your arms straight in front of you to shoulder height.
4. Make small circles with your wrists to the right and then to the left.
5. Repeat a few times until your wrists feel looser.
6. Lower your arms back to your sides.

CHEST AND UPPER BACK STRETCH

Muscles worked: shoulders, chest, and upper back.
Main muscles: Trapezius, pectorals.

1. Sit or stand upright.
2. Place your hands on your shoulders and your elbows out to the sides.
3. Touch your elbows together in front of your chest.
4. Swing your elbows out again and bring your shoulder blades together.
5. Repeat until your chest and upper back muscles feel looser.

SIMPLE KNEE PULLER

Muscles worked: Lower back and back of the thigh.
Main muscles: Hamstrings, erector spinor.

1. Sit straight.
2. Bend over and pull your knee towards your chest holding it with both hands.
3. Try to touch the knee with the forehead or as close as possible.
4. Hold the position for about 10 seconds and lower the knee again.
5. Repeat with the other leg.

CALF STRETCH

Muscles worked: Calves.
Main muscles: Gastrocnemius.

1. Stand up straight and hold onto something for support.
2. Pass your right leg back and make sure your heel is pressed against the floor.
3. Slightly bend your front leg, making it lean forward.
4. Hold for about 10 seconds.
5. Repeat with the other leg.

Tip: If you can't feel the stretch, move your back leg a little further back.

HAMSTRING STRETCH

Muscles worked: Back of the thigh.
Main muscles: Hamstrings.

1. Sit upright in a chair or on the floor.
2. With a towel, place it under your foot and straighten your leg lifting it off the floor.
3. Gently pull the ends of the towel toward you by flexing the foot toward you.
4. Hold for about 10 seconds. Put your foot back on the floor and repeat with the other leg.
5. If it is easy for you, sit on the floor with one leg stretched out in front and reach your toes.

QUADRICEPS STRETCH

Muscles worked: Front of the thigh.
Main muscles: Quadriceps.

1. Stand up straight and hold onto something for support.
2. Hold onto your right ankle with your right hand.
3. Bring your foot to your butt keeping your knees together.
4. Hold for 10 seconds.
5. Drop your foot on the ground and repeat with the other leg.

Frequently Asked Questions

What Do I Need for the Exercise Sessions?

To Be Convinced

Try the exercise for a period of 3 months. A single exercise session alone will not help, but as time goes on, you will begin to feel the benefit. Consider exercise as part of your treatment, along with your diet and medications.

Persistence

There will be times when you will miss your exercise sessions for various reasons, including hospitalizations. Do not give up! Start over. If your free time has made you less fit, start from that lower threshold and your fitness will soon improve again. There will be good days and bad days. If some days you feel very tired, you can exercise for a shorter period of time. Even 10 minutes is better than nothing!

Clothes and Shoes

You don't need fancy or expensive sportswear to exercise. Wear comfortable shoes (no high heels!) And clothes that aren't too tight. If you have multiple layers of lightweight clothing, you can remove or add a few as needed.

How Can I Make Exercise Part of My Busy Life?

Anyone can incorporate some exercise into their life; it is surprisingly easy. Remember: it will really help you, so it's worth making it a priority.

Some suggestions:

- **At home:** When the TV is on, do some stretching and resistance exercises or even cardiovascular exercises, like riding a stationary bike.
- **On the way to work:** Get off the bus one stop earlier or find a parking spot further away and walk 10 minutes to the office.
- **At work:** Take a walk during your lunch break. A brisk walk can help you feel refreshed and allow you to work better in the afternoon. Another opportunity to get in shape is to take the stairs instead of the elevator.
- **To get things done:** Walk or bike to the stores and maybe take the groceries home. Take the opportunity to work in the garden.
- **In your spare time:** Have your family or friends exercise with you; It's good for them too! Take out a ball or a Frisbee and offer to play with the children or ride a bike or walk.

Are There Times When I Shouldn't Exercise?

Yes. Talk to your doctor before you start exercising:

- If you have any change in your medicine prescription.
- If you are on dialysis and your dialysis schedule has changed.
- If you have any problems with your joints or bones that get worse with exercise.
- If you have a fever.
- If you have any change in your physical condition.
- If the weather is very hot and humid or very cold (unless you are exercising somewhere with air conditioning/heating).

What Are the Signs That I Should Stop Exercising?

Stop your exercise immediately if you notice any of the following symptoms during an exercise session:

1. You feel pain in your chest.
2. You notice a fast or irregular heartbeat.
3. You feel sick.
4. Feel cramps in the legs.
5. You feel light-headed or dizzy.

Considerations Before Starting to Exercise

Exercise doesn't have to be for athletes! It is never too late to start reaping the benefits of exercise, no matter what age or disability you think you have.

- If you are new to exercise, start lightly and gradually increase your activity level. Start with 10 minutes and build up to 30 minutes over time. Brisk walking is an ideal activity to start with.
- Set goals. Setting realistic goals can help you stay motivated to exercise. However, make goals clear and be careful not to set goals too high; you may lose your enthusiasm if you cannot achieve them.
- Keeping an exercise journal can be a good motivational tool by helping you keep track of your progress.
- Remember to include muscle strengthening exercises. You should do resistance exercises at least twice a week, although these should not be on consecutive days.
- Use daily activities as part of your exercise routine, this can count towards your 30 minutes per day. Consider a brisk walk to stores or work instead of taking the bus or car; If you can, take the stairs instead of an elevator or try to reduce the amount of time you are inactive (time spent sitting watching TV, etc.). There are many ways to do this, these are just a few!
- Find an exercise you can enjoy! If one type of activity or exercise gets boring, try switching to another. If you enjoy it, you are more likely to keep up.

If you need more advice, talk to the doctors, nurses, or other members of the clinical team that you see regularly.

LEARN HOW TO COOK

Spend Time on the Art of Cooking

Without a doubt, cooking is not something that you learn overnight. It is something that takes a lot of practice and hours of dedication. But learning to cook will allow you to have total control over what you consume, how much you consume it, and when you consume it. Many people (either due to lack of initiative, fatigue, or lack of time) go to fast food outlets or buy processed food in supermarkets, which leads to establishing unhealthy eating habits that are getting worse and worse.

Therefore, cooking is the best tool you have at your fingertips to be able to decide the ingredients of your meals and maintain strict control of your diet.

- Buy fresh food often. Sodium (a part of salt) is added to many prepared or packaged foods that you buy at the grocery store or at restaurants.
- Cook foods from scratch instead of eating prepared foods, "fast" foods, frozen dinners, and high-sodium canned foods. When you prepare your own food, you control what it contains.
- Use sodium-free spices, herbs, and seasonings instead of salt.
- Check the Nutrition Facts label on food packages for sodium. A daily value of 20 percent or more means that the food is high in sodium.
- Try low-sodium versions of frozen dinners and other prepared meals.
- Rinse canned vegetables, beans, meats, and fish with water before eating.

An important function of the kidneys is to remove waste and excess fluid from your body through urine. They too:

- Balance the minerals in your body, such as salt and potassium.
- Balance your body fluids.
- Produce hormones that affect the way other organs work.

A kidney-friendly diet is a way of eating that helps protect the kidneys from further damage. You will need to limit some foods and fluids so that other fluids and minerals like electrolytes don't build up in your body. At the same time, you'll need to make sure you get the right balance of protein, calories, vitamins, and minerals. If you are in the early stages of CKD, there may be few, if any, limits on what you can eat. But as your disease worsens, you will have to be more careful about what you inject into your body. Your doctor may suggest that you work with a dietitian to choose foods that are gentle on your kidneys.

This mineral is found naturally in many foods. It is most common in table salt. Sodium affects your blood pressure. It also helps maintain the water balance in your body. Healthy kidneys keep sodium levels under control. But if you have CKD, sodium, and extra fluids build up in your body. This can cause a number of problems, such as swollen ankles, high blood pressure, shortness of breath, and fluid buildup around the heart and lungs. You should aim for less than 2 grams of sodium in your daily diet. Follow these simple steps to reduce sodium in your diet:

- Avoid table salt and seasonings that are high in sodium (soy sauce, sea salt, garlic salt, etc.).
- Cook at home: Most fast foods are high in sodium.
- Try new spices and herbs instead of salt.
- Stay away from packaged foods, if possible. They are usually high in sodium.
- Read labels when shopping for and choosing foods low in sodium.
- Rinse canned foods (vegetables, beans, meats, and fish) with water before serving.

You need these minerals to keep your bones healthy and strong. When your kidneys are healthy, they get rid of phosphorus that you don't need. But if you have CKD, your phosphorus levels can get too high. This puts you at risk for heart disease. What's more, your calcium levels begin to drop. To compensate, your body extracts it from your bones. This can weaken them and make them easier to break. If you have late-stage CKD, your doctor may recommend that you eat no more than 1,000 milligrams (mg) of the mineral phosphorus per day. You can do this as follows:

- Choose foods low in phosphorus (look for "PHOS" on the label).
- Eat more fresh fruits and vegetables.
- Choose corn and rice cereals.
- Drink light-colored sodas.
- Reduce meat, poultry, and fish.
- Limit dairy products.

Foods high in calcium also tend to be high in phosphorus. Your doctor may suggest that you cut down on foods high in calcium. Low-phosphorous dairy foods include:

- Brie or Swiss cheese.
- Regular or low-fat cream cheese or sour cream.
- Sorbet.

WHAT SHOULD I EAT?

Foods You Should Eat

Next, a series of foods that are very beneficial for all those with kidney disease will be listed.

- **Red bell peppers:** Red bell peppers are low in potassium and high in flavor, but that's not the only reason they are perfect for the kidney diet. These tasty greens are also an excellent source of vitamin C and vitamin A, as well as vitamin B6, folate, and fiber. Red bell peppers are good for you because they contain lycopene, an antioxidant that protects against certain cancers. Eat raw red bell peppers with salsa as a snack or appetizer, or mix them with tuna or chicken salad. You can also roast bell peppers and use them as a topping on sandwiches or lettuce salads, chop them to make an omelet, add them to grilled skewers, or stuff bell peppers with ground turkey or beef and bake them as a main dish.

- **Cabbage:** A cruciferous vegetable, cabbage is packed with phytochemicals, chemical compounds in fruits or vegetables that break down free radicals before they can cause harm. Many phytochemicals are also known to protect against and fight cancer, in addition to promoting cardiovascular health. High in vitamin K, vitamin C, and fiber, cabbage is also a good source of vitamin B6 and folate. Low in potassium and inexpensive, it is an affordable supplement to the kidney diet. Raw cabbage is a great addition to the dialysis diet as coleslaw or fish taco dressing. You can steam, microwave, or boil it, add butter or cream cheese plus pepper or caraway seeds and serve as a garnish. Cabbage rolls made with turkey make a great appetizer, and if you feel like it, you can stuff a cabbage with ground beef and bake it for a tasty meal full of nutrients.

- **Cauliflower:** Another cruciferous vegetable, cauliflower is high in vitamin C and a good source of folate and fiber. It's also packed with indoles, glucosinolates, and thiocyanates, compounds that help the liver neutralize toxic substances that could damage cell membranes and DNA. Serve it raw as a crudité with sauce, add to a salad, or steam or boil and season with spices like turmeric, curry powder, pepper, and herb seasonings. You can also make a dairy-free white sauce, pour it over the cauliflower, and bake until tender. You can combine cauliflower with pasta or even puree cauliflower as a dialysis diet replacement for mashed potatoes.

- **Garlic:** Garlic helps prevent plaque formation on teeth, lowers cholesterol, and reduces inflammation. Buy it fresh, bottled, minced, or powdered, and add it to meat, vegetable, or pasta dishes. You can also roast a head of garlic and spread it on bread. Garlic provides a delicious flavor and garlic powder is an excellent substitute for garlic salt in the dialysis diet.

- **Onions:** Onions, a member of the Allium family and a basic flavoring in many cooked dishes, contain sulfur compounds that give it its pungent odor. But in addition to making some people cry, onions are also rich in flavonoids, especially quercetin, a powerful antioxidant that works to reduce heart disease and protects against many cancers. Onions are low in potassium and a good source of chromium, a mineral that helps with the metabolism of carbohydrates, fats, and proteins. Try using several varieties of onions, including white, brown, red, and others. Eat raw onions in burgers, sandwiches, and salads, cook them and use them as a caramelized topping, or fry them in onion rings. Include onions in recipes like Italian beef with peppers and onions.

- **Apples:** Apples are known to lower cholesterol, prevent constipation, protect against heart disease, and reduce the risk of cancer. High in fiber and anti-inflammatory compounds, an apple a day can really keep the doctor away. Good news for people with kidney disease who already have their share of doctor visits. This Kidney Diet Winner can be combined with good-for-you food, onions, to make a one-of-a-kind apple and onion omelet. With apples, you can eat them raw, make baked apples, stew apples, turn them into applesauce, or drink them as apple juice or apple cider.

- **Lingonberries:** These spicy and flavorful berries are known to protect against bladder infections by preventing bacteria from sticking to the bladder wall. Similarly, blueberries also protect the stomach from ulcer-causing bacteria and protect the lining of the gastrointestinal (GI) tract, promoting GI health. Lingonberries have also been shown to protect against cancer and heart disease. Cranberry juice and cranberry sauce are the most widely consumed cranberry products. You can also add dried cranberries to salads or have them as a snack.

- **Blueberries:** Blueberries are rich in antioxidant phytonutrients called anthocyanidins, which give them their blue color, and are packed with natural compounds that reduce inflammation. Blueberries are a good source of vitamin C; manganese, a compound that keeps bones healthy; and fiber. They can also help protect the brain from some of the effects of aging. The antioxidants in blueberries and other berries have been shown to help slow bone breakdown in low-estrogen rats. Buy fresh, frozen, or dried blueberries and try them on cereal or, topped with whipped cream, in a fruit shake. You can also drink cranberry juice.

- **Raspberries:** Raspberries contain a phytonutrient called ellagic acid that helps neutralize free radicals in the body to prevent cell damage. They also contain flavonoids called anthocyanins, antioxidants that give them their red color. An excellent source of manganese, vitamin C, fiber, and folate, raspberries may have properties that inhibit cancer cell growth and tumor formation. Add raspberries to cereal or puree and sweeten to make a gravy. dessert or add to vinaigrette dressing.

- **Strawberries:** Strawberries are rich in two types of phenols: anthocyanins and ellagitannins. Anthocyanins are what give strawberries their red color and are powerful antioxidants that help protect the body's cellular structures and prevent oxidative damage. Strawberries are an excellent source of vitamin C and manganese and a very good source of fiber. They are known to provide heart protection as well as anti-cancer and anti-inflammatory components. Eat strawberries with cereal, smoothies, and salad, or slice them and serve fresh or top with whipped topping. For a more elaborate dessert, you can make a strawberry pudding or sorbet, or puree and sweeten it for dessert.

- **Cherries:** Cherries have been shown to reduce inflammation when eaten daily. They are also packed with antioxidants and phytochemicals that protect the heart. Eat fresh cherries as a snack or make a cherry sauce to go with lamb or pork. Cherry juice is another way to consume this tasty food.

- **Red grapes:** Red grapes contain various flavonoids that give them their reddish color. Flavonoids help protect against heart disease by preventing oxidation and reducing blood clots. Resveratrol, a flavonoid found in grapes, can also stimulate nitric oxide production which helps relax muscle cells in blood vessels to increase blood flow. These flavonoids also provide protection against cancer and prevent inflammation. Buy grapes with red or purple skin as their anthocyanin content is higher. Freeze to eat as a snack or to quench the thirst of those with a fluid restriction for the dialysis diet. Add grapes to a fruit salad or chicken salad. Try a unique kidney diet recipe for turkey kabobs that contain grapes. You can also drink them as grape juice.

- **Egg whites:** Egg whites are pure protein and provide the highest quality protein with all the essential amino acids. For the kidney diet, egg whites provide protein with less phosphorus than other protein sources such as egg yolk or meats. Buy powdered egg whites, fresh or pasteurized. Make an omelet or egg white sandwich, add pasteurized egg whites to shakes, make stuffed egg sandwiches, or add hard-boiled egg whites to tuna salad or garden salad for extra protein.

- **Fish:** Fish provides high-quality protein and contains anti-inflammatory fats called omega-3. The healthy fats in fish can help fight diseases like heart disease and cancer. Omega-3 also helps lower low-density lipoproteins or LDL cholesterol, which is bad cholesterol, and increase high-density lipoproteins or HDL cholesterol, which is good cholesterol. The American Heart Association and the American Diabetes Association recommend eating fish at least twice a week. The fish that are richest in omega-3 are albacore, herring, mackerel, rainbow trout, and salmon.

- **Olive oil:** Olive oil is a great source of oleic acid, an anti-inflammatory fatty acid. The monounsaturated fat in olive oil protects against oxidation. Olive oil is rich in polyphenols and antioxidant compounds that prevent inflammation and oxidation. Studies show that populations that use large amounts of olive oil instead of other oils have lower rates of heart disease and cancer. Buy virgin or extra virgin olive oil because they are higher in antioxidants. Use olive oil to make salad dressings, for cooking, for dipping bread, or for marinating vegetables. Talk to your kidney dietitian about incorporating these top 15 foods for a kidney diet into your healthy eating plan. Keep in mind that these foods are healthy for everyone, including family and friends who do not have kidney disease or are not on dialysis.

Foods to Avoid

Eat less salt/sodium. That is a good step for diabetes and really important for CKD. Over time, the kidneys lose the ability to control sodium and water balance. Less sodium in your diet will help lower blood pressure and reduce fluid build-up in your body, which is common in kidney disease. Focus on fresh comfort food and eat only small amounts of restaurant food and packaged food, which are usually high in sodium. Look for low sodium content (5% or less) on food labels.

In a week or two, you'll get used to having less salt in your food, especially if you boost the flavor with flavored herbs, spices, mustard, and vinegar. But don't use salt substitutes unless your doctor or dietitian says you can. Many are high in potassium, which you may need to limit. Depending on the stage of your kidney disease, you may also need to reduce potassium, phosphorus, and protein in your diet. Many foods that are part of a typical healthy diet may not be suitable for a CKD diet. Phosphorous is a mineral that keeps bones strong and other parts of the body healthy. Your kidneys cannot remove extra phosphorus from your blood very well. Too much weakens the bones and can damage the blood vessels, eyes, and heart. Meat, dairy, beans, nuts, whole wheat bread, and dark-colored sodas are high in phosphorus. Phosphorus is also added to many packaged foods. The right level of potassium keeps your nerves and muscles working well. With CKD, too much potassium can build up in the blood and cause serious heart problems. Oranges, potatoes, tomatoes, whole wheat bread, and many other foods are high in potassium. Apples, carrots, and white bread are lower in potassium. Your doctor may prescribe a potassium chelator, a medicine that helps your body get rid of excess potassium. Get the right amount of protein. More protein than you need makes your kidneys work harder and can make CKD worse. But very little is not healthy either. Both animal and plant foods have protein. Your dietitian can help you determine the correct combination and amount of protein to eat.

CONTROLLING BLOOD PRESSURE AND DIABETES

What Nutrients Are Needed to Regulate Them?

After having carried out the corresponding studies, your family doctor together with other specialists will be the ones to tell you which nutrients you should ingest in your daily diet and which are the best foods to provide them on a day-to-day basis.

The Role of Proteins in Kidney Disease

We all need protein in our diet every day. Proteins, carbohydrates, and fats are the three sources of fuel (calories) in the food we eat. Protein is used to build muscle and fight infection.

How do you know how much protein you need every day? Protein needs vary based on your age, gender, and general health. The recommended daily allowance (RDA) for protein in healthy adults is 0.8 grams of protein per kilogram of desirable body weight per day. So for a 150-pound person (divide by 2.2 to get 68 kilograms and then multiply by 0.8), that's 55 grams of protein a day. For someone who weighs 120 pounds, that would be 44 grams of protein per day. If we eat more protein than our body can use in a day, it becomes a source of excess calories, which can lead to weight gain. Protein by-products are removed from the body by the kidneys, which filter them into the urine.

For someone with declining kidney function, the byproducts of protein breakdown in the body can accumulate in the blood rather than be eliminated. Many studies suggest that limiting the amount of protein in the diet can delay the loss of kidney function. It is important that a kidney doctor (nephrologist) and a renal dietitian help plan the amount and type of protein sources to provide in your diet, even in the earliest stages of kidney disease, so that the function of kidney disease can be closely monitored in case changes in diet and medications are necessary.

The protein sources in our diet come from animal and plant sources. Animal sources of protein are considered "complete" or "high-quality" proteins, as they provide all essential amino acids (the building blocks of protein). Animal sources of protein vary in their amount of fat, with fatty cuts of red meat and whole-milk dairy products and eggs being the highest in saturated fat (least healthy for the heart). Fish, poultry, and low-fat or fat-free dairy products are the lowest in saturated fat.

An "incomplete" or "lower quality" protein source is one that is low in one or more of the essential amino acids. Plant sources like beans, lentils, nuts, peanut butter, seeds, and whole grains are examples of incomplete protein. The good news is that if you consume a combination of these incomplete proteins on the same day, they can provide adequate amounts of all the essential amino acids. Vegetarians can meet their protein needs with careful planning. For example, the combination of kidney beans and rice or peanut butter in whole wheat bread forms a complete protein. Another advantage of plant proteins is that they are low in saturated fat and high in fiber.

CONVERSION TABLES

Oven Temperatures

Fahrenheit (°F)	Celsius (°C)
250 °F	120 °C
300 °F	150 °C
325 °F	165 °C
350 °F	180 °C
375 °F	190 °C
400 °F	200 °C
425 °F	220 °C
450 °F	230 °C

Volume Equivalences (Liquids)

US Equivalences	Conversion
1/8 teaspoon	0.5 mL
1/4 teaspoon	1 mL
1/2 teaspoon	2 mL
2/3 teaspoon	4 mL
1 teaspoon	5 mL
1 tablespoon	15 mL
1/4 cup	59 mL
1/3 cup	79 mL
1/2 cup	118 mL
2/3 cup	156 mL
3/4 cup	177 mL
1 cup	235 mL
2 cup	475 mL
3 cup	700 mL
4 cup	1 L
1/2 gallon	2 L
1 gallon	4 L

Weight Equivalences

US Equivalences	Conversion
1/2 ounce	15 g
1 ounce	30 g
2 ounces	60 g
4 ounces	115 g
8 ounces	225 g
12 ounces	340 g
16 ounces or 1 pound	455 g

BREAKFAST

1. CEREAL SNACK MIX WITH NO-SALT SEASONING

Servings: 5
Ingredients:

6 tablespoons butter (unsalted)
3 tablespoons Mrs. Dash® Onion & Herb Seasoning Mix
8 cups Crispix Cereal
2 cups unsalted pretzels
2 cups oyster crackers

Instructions:

1. Preheat oven to 250 degrees Fahrenheit.
2. On a shallow baking sheet, melt the butter.
3. Combine seasonings and stir to combine. Toss the cereal, pretzels, and oyster crackers into the butter mixture and toss to coat.
4. Bake for 60 minutes, stirring every 15 minutes after removing the pan from the oven.

> **Nutritional value:**
> - Energy value: 244 Kcal
> - Proteins: 26 g
> - Carbohydrates: 3 g
> - Fiber: 2 g
> - Sugar: 4 g
> - Sodium: 2 g
> - Fats: 12 g
>   ***Of which:***
>   - Saturated: 3 g
>   - Monounsaturated: 6 g
>   - Polyunsaturated: 2 g
> - Cholesterol: 135 mg

2. EASY SUMMER FRUIT DIP

Servings: 2
Ingredients:

8 oz. low-fat cream cheese
7 oz. marshmallow cream

Instructions:

- Cream cheese should soften.
- Using an electric mixer, combine the marshmallow and cream cheese well.
- Serve with fruits for dipping that are good for the kidneys.

> **Nutritional value:**
> - Energy value: 124 Kcal
> - Proteins: 15 g
> - Carbohydrates: 12 g
> - Fiber: 5 g
> - Sugar: 6 g
> - Sodium: 8 g
> - Fats: 12 g
>   ***Of which:***
>   - Saturated: 7 g
>   - Monounsaturated: 3 g
>   - Polyunsaturated: 1 g
>
> Cholesterol: 128 mg

3. APPLE TOAST

Servings: 5
Ingredients:

2 flour tortillas, 6-inch size, use non-stick cooking spray
1 teaspoon sugar (granulated)
A quarter teaspoon pumpkin pie spice
2 apples, medium
1 tablespoon of sugar (brown)
1/2 gallon of apple juice
1 cup of water
1 tablespoon currants (dried)
1 teaspoon powdered sugar, sifted

Instructions:

1. Preheat the oven to 400 degrees Fahrenheit.
2. Tortillas should be cut in half. Toss tortillas with nonstick cooking spray and place them on a baking sheet.
3. Combine granulated sugar and 1/4 teaspoon pumpkin pie spice in a small bowl. Toss toppings over tortilla halves. Preheat oven to 350 degrees Fahrenheit and bake for 10 minutes or until crisp.
4. On a wire rack, cool completely.
5. Apples should be peeled, cored, and sliced.
6. Preheat a medium nonstick skillet over medium heat with a light coating of cooking spray. Cook and stir for about 10 minutes, or until golden brown, add apples, brown sugar, and the remaining 1/2 teaspoon pumpkin pie spice.
7. Combine apple juice, water, and currants in a mixing bowl. Cook for another 20 minutes, stirring occasionally, or until the apples have caramelized and the liquid has evaporated.
8. Place half a tortilla on a dessert plate and top with 1/2 cup apple mix. Sprinkle with powdered sugar, if desired.
9. Serve immediately.

> **Nutritional value:**
> - Energy value: 100 Kcal
> - Proteins: 8 g
> - Carbohydrates: 12g
> - Fiber: 9 g
> - Sugar: 3 g
> - Sodium: 2 g
> - Fats: 12 g
>   ***Of which:***
>   - Saturated: 6 g
>   - Monounsaturated: 4 g
>   - Polyunsaturated: 1 g
> - Cholesterol: 80 mg

4. ACAI BERRY SMOOTHIE BOWL

Servings: 2
Ingredients:

1 tablespoon of unsweetened frozen acai
1 cup frozen mixed berries, unsweetened
3/4 cup plain low-fat Greek yogurt (2% fat)
1 teaspoon of chia seeds
1/2 cup of rice milk without sugar, original, classic
2 tablespoons of raspberry juice
2 tablespoons of blueberries
1 pear, fresh

Instructions:

1. Remove the frozen acai puree from the package and mash it.

2. In a blender, combine acai, frozen mixed berries, Greek yogurt, chia seeds, and rice milk.
3. Blend until completely smooth. You should be able to eat it with a spoon if the consistency is thick enough.
4. Divide mixed batter evenly between two bowls.
5. Top with raspberries, blueberries, and chopped pear.

> **Nutritional value:**
> - Energy value: 227 Kcal
> - Proteins: 5 g
> - Carbohydrates: 7 g
> - Fiber: 5 g
> - Sugar: 3 g
> - Sodium: 2 g
> - Fat: 9 g
>   - *Of which:*
>   - o   Saturated: 7 g
>   - o   Monounsaturated: 1 g
>   - o   Polyunsaturated: 1 g
> - Cholesterol: 100 mg

5. BELGIAN WAFFLES

Servings: 2
Ingredients:

2 large eggs
2 cups of cake flour
3/4 teaspoon of baking soda
3/4 cup sour cream
3/4 cup 1% skim milk
2 teaspoons of vanilla extract
4 tablespoons unsalted butter
2 tablespoons granulated sugar
6 tablespoons powdered sugar

Instructions:
1. Heat waffle iron. In a bowl, mix together the cake flour and baking soda and set aside. Separate the whites and yolks. Collectively beat the egg yolks, sour cream, milk, and vanilla extract. Melt the butter and then mix with the added sour cream.
2. In a single bowl, beat the egg whites with a hand mixer on medium speed until soft peaks form, about 3 minutes. Add the granulated sugar to the egg whites and keep to beat until stiff peaks form, for about 3 to 4 more minutes.
3. Beat sour cream combination into flour mixture until just combined. Gently fold in beaten egg whites until the combination is clean; now, don't over mix.
4. Add about half of the batter to the waffle iron, close, and cook dinner for about 3 minutes. Serve the waffles with icing sugar. Other recommended toppings consist of clean berries, whipped cream, jam, or syrup.

> **Nutritional value:**
> - Energy value: 153 Kcal
> - Proteins: 7 g
> - Carbohydrates: 16 g
> - Fiber: 7 g
> - Sugar: 5 g
> - Sodium: 2 g
> - Fats: 13 g
>   - *Of which:*
>   - o   Saturated: 4 g
>   - o   Monounsaturated: 6 g
>   - o   Polyunsaturated: 2 g
> Cholesterol: 115 mg

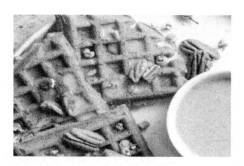

6. APPLE CINNAMON MAPLE GRANOLA

Servings: 3
Ingredients:

3 cups of puffed rice cereal
3 cups of old oats
3/4 ounce package of baked apple chips
1/2 of sugared dried cranberries
1/2 teaspoon ground cinnamon
1 teaspoon of nutmeg
1/4 cup coconut oil, melted
1/4 cup of 100% natural maple syrup
1 ½ teaspoons vanilla extract
1/2 cup unsweetened applesauce

Instructions:
1. Preheat oven to 275 degrees Fahrenheit. Line 2 large baking sheets with parchment paper.
2. Combine dry items in a large bowl.
3. Combine wet ingredients in a small bowl.
4. Pour wet ingredients into the dry ingredients container. Mix very well to cover dry items.
5. Divide mixture among 2 baking sheets.
6. Bake for 50 minutes to an hour, changing baking sheets position (move baking sheets from upper rack to lower rack) halfway through baking.

> **Nutritional value:**
> - Energy value: 192 Kcal
> - Proteins: 19 g
> - Carbohydrates: 15 g
> - Fiber: 7 g
> - Sugar: 3 g
> - Sodium: 3 g
> - Fats: 10 g
>   - *Of which:*
>   - o   - Saturated: 5 g
>   - o   - Monounsaturated: 3 g
>   - o   - Polyunsaturated: 1 g
> - Cholesterol: 127 mg

7. BREAKFAST CASSEROLE

Servings: 5
Ingredients:

8 ounces low-fat red meat sausage
8 ounces cream cheese
1 cup of 1% low-fat milk
4 slices of white bread, diced or broken
5 huge eggs
1/2 teaspoon of dry mustard
1/2 teaspoon of dried onion flakes

Instructions:
1. Preheat oven to 325 degrees Fahrenheit.
2. Crumble the sausage and cook it in a medium saucepan.
3. Mix final substances, in addition to bread, in the moneylender.
4. Add cooked sausage to the mixture.
5. Place bread crumbs in greased 9x9" casserole. Pour the sausage mixture over the bread.

6. Bake for 55 minutes or until set.
7. Cut into 9 portions and serve.

> **Nutritional value:**
> - Energy value: 260 Kcal
> - Proteins: 5 g
> - Carbohydrates: 16 g
> - Fiber: 4 g
> - Sugar: 4 g
> - Sodium: 5 g
> - Fat: 18 g
>   **Of which:**
>   - - Saturated: 5 g
>   - - Monounsaturated: 7 g
>   - - Polyunsaturated: 4 g
>
> Cholesterol: 119 mg

8. APPLE CINNAMON FRENCH TOAST STRATA

Servings: 5
Ingredients:

1 pound cinnamon raisin bread
8 ounces cream cheese
1 half of medium apples
6 tablespoons unsalted butter
1 teaspoon of ground cinnamon
8 large eggs
1 ¼ cup cream
1 ¼ cup almond milk, unsweetened
1/4 cup pancake syrup

Instructions:
1. Cut the bread and cream cheese into cubes. Peel and dice the apples. Melt the butter.
2. Coat a 9x13" baking dish with nonstick cooking spray. Place half of the cubed bread on the bottom of the plate. Sprinkle the cream cheese cubes over the bread and make a pinnacle with the apples. Sprinkle cinnamon over the apples and sprinkle with the remaining bread.
3. In a large bowl, whisk the eggs with half the cream and half, the almond milk, melted butter, and pancake syrup. Pour the aggregate over the bread. Put on a plastic wrap baking dish and press down to soak all pieces. Refrigerate for at least 2 hours or in a single day.
4. Preheat oven to 325 degrees Fahrenheit.
5. Bake the strata for 50 minutes, then let it rest for 10 minutes before serving. Cut lightly into squares for 12 servings.
6. Top with pancake syrup, sugar syrup, jelly, or cinnamon/raspberry applesauce if you prefer.

> **Nutritional value:**
> - Energy value: 192 Kcal
> - Proteins: 19 g
> - Carbohydrates: 15 g
> - Fiber: 7 g
> - Sugar: 3 g
> - Sodium: 3 g
> - Fats: 10 g
>   **Of which:**
>   - - Saturated: 5 g
>   - - Monounsaturated: 3 g
>   - - Polyunsaturated: 1 g
> - Cholesterol: 127 mg

9. BLUEBERRY SMOOTHIE BOWL

Servings: 1
Ingredients:

1 cup frozen blueberries
2 scoops of whey protein powder
1/4 cup plain, nonfat Greek yogurt
1/3 cup unsweetened vanilla almond milk
2 medium strawberries
5 raspberries
1 tablespoon high-fiber cereal
2 teaspoons of grated coconut

Instructions:
1. Place the blueberries in a blender and blend over low heat for 1 minute.
2. Add protein powder, yogurt, and almond milk. Blend until smooth to serve. Scrape the sides of the blender.
3. Pour the mixture into a bowl.
4. Top with sliced strawberries, clean raspberries, high-fiber cereal, and coconut flakes. Add honey or sugar if you prefer.

> **Nutritional value:**
> - Energy value: 280 Kcal
> - Proteins: 8 g
> - Carbohydrates: 14 g
> - Fiber: 7 g
> - Sugar: 5 g
> - Sodium: 2 g
> - Fats: 13 g
>   **Of which:**
>   - - Saturated: 4 g
>   - - Monounsaturated: 6 g
>   - - Polyunsaturated: 2 g
>
> Cholesterol: 2mg

10. DILLY SCRAMBLED EGGS

Servings: 1
Ingredients:

2 large eggs
1/8 teaspoon black pepper
1 teaspoon dried dill
1 tablespoon crumbled goat cheese

Instructions:
1. Beat the eggs in a bowl; Pour them into a nonstick skillet over medium heat.
2. Add black pepper and dill to the eggs.
3. Cook until eggs are scrambled.
4. Top with crumbled goat cheese before serving.

> **Nutritional value:**
> - Energy value: 153 Kcal
> - Proteins: 7 g
> - Carbohydrates: 16 g
> - Fiber: 7 g
> - Sugar: 5 g
> - Sodium: 2 g
> - Fats: 13 g
>   **Of which:**
>   - - Saturated: 4 g
>   - - Monounsaturated: 6 g
>   - - Polyunsaturated: 2 g
>
> Cholesterol: 115mg

BRUNCH

11. COLD VEGGIE PIZZA SANDWICHES

Servings: 5

Ingredients:

Half-moon roll dough (16 ounces)
Half a cup of sour cream
1 cup of whipped cream cheese
2 tablespoons Ranch Salad Dressing (low fat)
1/4 teaspoon of garlic powder
1 cup broccoli florets
1 medium carrot
1/2 cucumber (medium)
1/2 cup red onion
1/2 cup of cherry tomatoes

Instructions:

1. Preheat the oven to 350 degrees Fahrenheit. With nonstick cooking spray, line 13x9x2" baking pan.
2. To make a single flat dough surface, spread out both packages of crescent rolls on the baking sheet. Preheat oven to 350 degrees Fahrenheit and bake for 10–15 minutes. Let cool 10–15 minutes.
3. Beat cream cheese and sour cream in a bowl until smooth. Combine ranch dressing and garlic powder in a mixing bowl. Using a spatula, spread the mixture evenly over the base.
4. The broccoli, carrot, cucumber, and onion should be chopped. Cherry tomatoes can be cut in half.
5. On top of the cream cheese mixture, place the chopped vegetables.
6. Cover pizza with plastic wrap and keep refrigerated until ready to serve. For 20 bits, make 4 even vertical cuts and 5 horizontal cuts.

Nutritional value:
- Energy value: 260 Kcal
- Proteins: 5 g
- Carbohydrates: 16 g
- Fiber: 4 g
- Sugar: 4 g
- Sodium: 5 g
- Fat: 18 g
  Of which:
  - Saturated: 5 g
  - Monounsaturated: 7 g
  - Polyunsaturated: 4 g
- Cholesterol: 119 mg

12. DILL NIBBLES

Servings: 4

Ingredients:

28 ounces of rice cereal
1/2 teaspoon of garlic powder
1 1/2 tablespoons dried dill
1/2 cup of grated Parmesan cheese
1 teaspoon Worcestershire sauce
1/2 cup of unsalted butter

Instructions:

1. Preheat the oven to 250 degrees Fahrenheit.
2. Fill a large baking dish halfway with cereal.
3. In a saucepan, melt the butter over medium-low heat.

4. Mix together the butter, garlic powder, dill, Parmesan cheese, and Worcestershire sauce.
5. Melt the butter in a saucepan. 1/4 of the butter mixture should be poured over the cereal in the skillet and mixed to coat the cereal. 15 minutes in the oven.
6. Remove the cereal from the oven and add about 1/4 of the butter mixture on top, mixing well. Cook for another 15 minutes in the oven.
7. Repeat steps 6 and 7 until all of the butter mixture has been added and the cereal has cooked for an hour until crisp.

Nutritional value:
- Energy value: 192 Kcal
- Proteins: 19 g
- Carbohydrates: 15 g
- Fiber: 7 g
- Sugar: 3 g
- Sodium: 3 g
- Fats: 10 g
  Of which:
  - Saturated: 5 g
  - Monounsaturated: 3 g
  - Polyunsaturated: 1 g
- Cholesterol: 127 mg

13. APPLE AND ONION OMELET

Servings: 2

Ingredients:

3 large eggs
1/4 cup 1% low-fat milk
1 tablespoon of water
1/8 teaspoon black pepper
1 tablespoon butter
3/4 cup sweet onion
1 huge apple
2 tablespoons grated cheddar cheese

Instructions:

1. Preheat the oven to 400 degrees Fahrenheit.
2. Peel and core the apple. Cut the apple and onion into thin slices.
3. Beat the eggs with the milk, water, and pepper in a small bowl; set aside.
4. Over medium heat, melt the butter in a small ovenproof skillet.
5. Add onion and apple to skillet and sauté until onion turns translucent, for about 5 to 6 minutes.
6. Spread the onion and apple mixture calmly into the pan.
7. Pour the egg mixture lightly into the skillet and cook the dinner over medium heat until they start to set. Sprinkle the cheddar cheese over the pinnacle. Transfer skillet to oven and bake until center is set, about 10 to 12 minutes.
8. Cut the tortilla in half and slide each half onto a plate. Serve right now.

Nutritional value:
- Energy value: 153 Kcal
- Proteins: 21g
- Carbohydrates: 16 g
- Fiber: 7 g
- Sugar: 7 g
- Sodium: 2 g
- Fats: 13 g

Of which:
- o   - Saturated: 4 g
- o   - Monounsaturated: 6 g
- o   - Polyunsaturated: 2 g

Cholesterol: 115mg

14. BREAKFAST BURRITO

Servings: 2
Ingredients:

Non-stick cooking spray
4 eggs
3 tablespoons Ortega® chilies, diced
1/4 teaspoon ground cumin
1/2 teaspoon of hot sauce
2 flour tortillas

Instructions:

1. Spray a medium-size skillet with nonstick cooking spray and heat over medium heat.

2. In a bowl, beat the eggs with chili peppers, cumin, and hot sauce. Pour the eggs into the skillet and cook the dinner and stir for 1 to 2 minutes until the eggs are set.

3. Heat the tortillas for 20 seconds in the microwave or in a separate skillet over medium heat. Place half of the eggs on each tortilla and roll burrito style.

Nutritional value:
- • Energy value: 260 Kcal
- • Proteins: 21g
- • Carbohydrates: 16 g
- • Fiber: 7 g
- • Sugar: 7 g
- • Sodium: 2 g
- • Fats: 13 g
  - **Of which:**
    - o   - Saturated: 4 g
    - o   - Monounsaturated: 6 g
    - o   - Polyunsaturated: 2 g

Cholesterol: 119mg

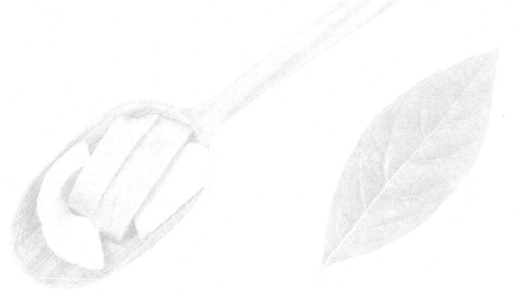

34

SIDE DISHES AND SNACKS

15. STUFFED EGGS FOR PARTIES

Servings: 4
Ingredients:

24 quail eggs
1/2 cup of mayonnaise
1 tablespoon mustard (optional)
1 teaspoon cayenne pepper
1 teaspoon paprika

Instructions:

1. Cook the eggs for 15 to 20 minutes at a low temperature.
2. Let the eggs cool for 1 hour.
3. Remove the yolks by cutting the eggs in half lengthwise.
4. Mix the egg yolks, mayonnaise, vinegar, and peppers well.
5. Fill the egg white halves halfway with the yolk and paprika mixture.

> **Nutritional value:**
> - Energy value: 227 Kcal
> - Proteins: 5 g
> - Carbohydrates: 7 g
> - Fiber: 5 g
> - Sugar: 3 g
> - Sodium: 2 g
> - Fat: 9 g
>   - ***Of which:***
>   - Saturated: 7 g
>   - Monounsaturated: 1 g
>   - Polyunsaturated: 1 g
> - Cholesterol: 100 mg

16. STUFFED EGGS

Servings: 4
Ingredients:

2 chickens, large
2 tablespoons bell pepper (canned)
1/2 teaspoon mustard powder
2 tablespoons mayonnaise
1/4 teaspoon of black pepper
1/8 teaspoon paprika

Instructions:

1. Boil the eggs for a long time. Drain and let cool.
2. Remove the yolk from the eggs by peeling and cutting them lengthwise.
3. The pepper should be diced and combined with the yolk, dry mustard, mayonnaise, and black pepper.
4. In equal sections, place the mixture into the whites.
5. Paprika should be sprinkled over the eggs.

> **Nutritional value:**
> - Energy value: 260 Kcal
> - Proteins: 5 g
> - Carbohydrates: 16 g
> - Fiber: 4 g
> - Sugar: 4 g
> - Sodium: 5 g
> - Fat: 18 g
>   - ***Of which:***
>   - Saturated: 5 g
>   - Monounsaturated: 7 g
>   - Polyunsaturated: 4 g
> - Cholesterol: 119 mg

17. BREAD CUPS

Servings: 4
Ingredients:

24 slices white bread, thinly sliced
2 tablespoons canola oil
1 teaspoon warm chili oil
1 teaspoon garlic powder

Instructions:

1. Preheat the oven to 400 degrees Fahrenheit.
2. Cut the crust from the bread slices and roll them up with a rolling pin.
3. Spray a small cup muffin pan with nonstick cooking spray.
4. Press a slice of bread into each muffin pan and trim the edges with a knife.
5. Mix the oils and garlic powder. Brush each cup of bread with oil and bake for 10 to 12 minutes until crisp and golden.
6. Let cups cool before removing from muffin pan.

> **Nutritional value:**
> - Energy value: 153 Kcal
> - Proteins: 7 g
> - Carbohydrates: 16 g
> - Fiber: 7 g
> - Sugar: 5 g
> - Sodium: 2 g
> - Fats: 13 g
>   - ***Of which:***
>   - Saturated: 4 g
>   - Monounsaturated: 6 g
>   - Polyunsaturated: 2 g
> - Cholesterol: 115 mg

18. CRANBERRY ALMOND CELERY LOGS

Servings: 2
Ingredients:

4 sticks of celery (medium 8-inch)
4 tablespoons of cream cheese whipped with red berries
24 blueberries, dried and sweetened
12 almonds, whole, unsalted, dry roasted

Instructions:

1. Trim the ends of the celery sticks.
2. 1 tablespoon whipped cream cheese, stuffed on each rib of celery.
3. Each rib of celery should be cut into three sections.
4. 1 almond and 2 dried cranberries on top of each piece.
5. Refrigerate until ready to eat, covered.

> **Nutritional value:**
> - Energy value: 192 Kcal
> - Proteins: 19 g
> - Carbohydrates: 15 g
> - Fiber: 7 g
> - Sugar: 3 g
> - Sodium: 3 g
> - Fats: 10 g
>   - Of which:
>   - Saturated: 5 g
>   - Monounsaturated: 3 g
>   - Polyunsaturated: 1 g
> - Cholesterol: 127 mg

19. FLOUR TORTILLA CHIPS

Servings: 4
Ingredients:

6 flour tortillas, each 6" diameter
1/2 cup of canola oil

Instructions:

1. Each tortilla should be cut into 8 wedge-shaped pieces.
2. In a heavy skillet, heat enough oil to cover 1/4" of the skillet.
3. When the oil is sweet, add the tortilla pieces until golden and crisp.
4. Remove the fries from the skillet and drain them on paper towels.
5. Store the fries in an airtight bag until you are ready to eat them.

Nutritional value:
- Energy value: 134 Kcal
- Proteins: 8 g
- Carbohydrates: 7 g
- Fiber: 4 g
- Sugar: 3 g
- Sodium: 3 g
- Fats: 10 g
  - *Of which:*
    - o Saturated: 5 g
    - o Monounsaturated: 3 g
    - o Polyunsaturated: 1 g
- Cholesterol: 127 mg

20. ADDICTIVE PRETZELS

Servings: 4
Ingredients:

32 ounces packet of pretzels, no salt
1 cup canola oil
2 tablespoons Hidden Valley Ranch Dressing and Salad Seasoning
3 teaspoons garlic powder
3 teaspoons dill, dried

Instructions:

1. Preheat the oven to 175 degrees Fahrenheit.
2. Pretzels should be spread out on two 18x13" baking sheets so they are flat. Divide large pretzels into chunks or use whole bite-size pretzels.
3. Combine the garlic powder and dill in a bowl. Half of the seasonings should be reserved. Add the dry salad dressing mix and 3/4 cup canola oil to the other half. Pour evenly over pretzels and cover them with your hands to ensure an even layer.
4. Preheat the oven to 350 degrees Fahrenheit and bake for 1 hour, mixing the pretzels every 15 minutes.

5. Take the pretzels out of the oven and set them aside. Let cool before mixing with the remaining garlic powder, dill, and oil. Have fun!

Nutritional value:
- Energy value: 260 Kcal
- Proteins: 5 g
- Carbohydrates: 16 g
- Fiber: 4 g
- Sugar: 4 g
- Sodium: 5 g
- Fat: 18 g
  - *Of which:*
    - o Saturated: 5 g
    - o Monounsaturated: 7 g
    - o Polyunsaturated: 4 g
- Cholesterol: 119 mg

21. ROLL-UPS PARTY

Servings: 2
Ingredients:

4 ounces canned green chilies, chopped
1/2 teaspoon garlic powder
1/2 teaspoon of cumin
1/4 teaspoon chili powder
4 tablespoons green onion
8 ounces cream cheese
6 flour tortillas (8" diameter each)

Instructions:

1. Let the cream cheese melt in the refrigerator. The green onion must be cut into thin slices.
2. In a bowl, combine the green chilies, spices, and chives.
3. In a bowl, combine the softened cream cheese and sour cream.
4. Spread a thin layer of the cream cheese mixture on each tortilla, leaving about 1/4" of the edge exposed.
5. Make a jelly roll with the tortillas. To hold the rolls together, use a toothpick.
6. Refrigerate for at least an hour after covering.
7. Serve as a sandwich or appetizer by cutting the buns into 1" pieces.

Nutritional value:
- Energy value: 192 Kcal
- Proteins: 19 g
- Carbohydrates: 15 g
- Fiber: 7 g
- Sugar: 3 g
- Sodium: 3 g
- Fats: 10 g
  - *Of which:*
    - o Saturated: 5 g
    - o Monounsaturated: 3 g
    - o Polyunsaturated: 1 g
- Cholesterol: 127 mg

VEGETARIAN DISHES

22. ASPARAGUS CREAM

Servings: 2
Ingredients:

6 ounces cream cheese
8 ounces low sodium canned asparagus
1 tablespoon of mayonnaise
2 teaspoons shallots
1/4 cup of lemon juice

Instructions:

1. Let the cream cheese melt in the refrigerator.
2. Drain the asparagus well.
3. In a food processor, combine all ingredients and process until smooth. Transfer to a bowl, cover, and chill overnight.
4. Make sandwiches with the spread or serve with low sodium crackers.

> **Nutritional value:**
> - Energy value: 192 Kcal
> - Proteins: 19 g
> - Carbohydrates: 15 g
> - Fiber: 7 g
> - Sugar: 3 g
> - Sodium: 3 g
> - Fats: 4 g
>   **Of which:**
>   - Saturated: 5 g
>   - Monounsaturated: 3 g
>   - Polyunsaturated: 1 g
> Cholesterol: 110 mg

23. CORN BALLS AND CHEESE

Servings: 2
Ingredients:

2 cups frozen yellow corn
1 green chili
2 tablespoons coriander
1/2 cup cottage cheese
4 slices of white bread
1/2 cup all-purpose white flour
1 teaspoon cayenne pepper
1 teaspoon ground cumin
1 teaspoon coriander powder
1/4 teaspoon salt
2 quarts of olive oil

Instructions:

1. The corn must be thawed. The orange chili and cilantro should be finely chopped.
2. Combine the cheese and thawed corn on a mixing plate.
3. Soak the bread slices in water for a few minutes and then strain the excess water to let the bread dry. Combine this with the corn and cheese mixture. Combine rice, dried spices, and cilantro in a mixing bowl.
4. In a large skillet, heat the oil. Scoop the corn and cheese mixture into balls and place each ball in the hot oil. Cook until golden brown on both sides.
5. Remove the balls from the oil and drain the excess oil on a tray lined with a kitchen napkin.
6. Serve with Cilantro Chutney on the side.

> **Nutritional value:**
> - Energy value: 90 Kcal
> - Proteins: 19 g
> - Carbohydrates: 15 g
> - Fiber: 7 g
> - Sugar: 3 g
> - Sodium: 3 g
> - Fats: 9 g
>   **Of which:**
>   - Saturated: 5 g
>   - Monounsaturated: 3 g
>   - Polyunsaturated: 1 g
> Cholesterol: 12 mg

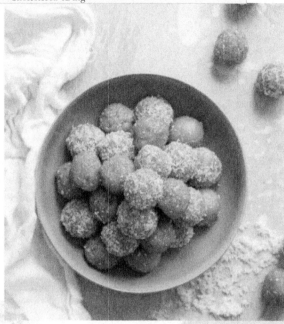

24. APPLE AND ONION OMELET

Servings: 2
Ingredients:

3 eggs (large)
1/4 cup of 1% skim milk
1 teaspoon of water
1/4 teaspoon of black pepper
1 tablespoon unsalted butter
3/4 cup sweet onion
1 large apple
2 tablespoons grated cheddar cheese

Instructions:

1. Preheat the oven to 400 degrees Fahrenheit.
2. Remove the core and peel the fruit. The apple and onion should be cut into thin slices.
3. In a small cup, combine the eggs, milk, water, and pepper; set aside.
4. In a small skillet, melt the butter over medium heat.
5. In a large skillet, sauté the onion and apple until the onion is translucent, about 5 to 6 minutes.
6. In the skillet, distribute the onion and apple mixture evenly.
7. Over medium heat, pour the egg mixture evenly into the skillet and cook until the edges begin to solidify. The cheddar cheese should be sprinkled on the end. Place the skillet in the oven and bake for 10 to 12 minutes, or until the center is set.
8. Cut the tortilla in half and place each half on its own plate. Serve immediately.

Nutritional value:
- Energy value: 260 Kcal
- Proteins: 5 g
- Carbohydrates: 16 g
- Fiber: 4 g
- Sugar: 4 g
- Sodium: 5 g
- Fat: 18 g
  - *Of which:*
    - Saturated: 5 g
    - Monounsaturated: 7 g
    - Polyunsaturated: 4 g

Cholesterol: 119 mg

25. ASPARAGUS AND CHEESE CREPE ROLLS WITH PARSLEY

Servings: 2
Ingredients:
12 asparagus
4 ounces cream cheese
1 package of parsley
1 teaspoon of lemon juice
1/2 teaspoon of black pepper
1/3 cup whole wheat flour
1/2 cup water
1/4 cup cream
1 egg
2 egg whites
4 tablespoons of butter

Instructions:
1. Steam the asparagus for 6 to 8 minutes.
2. Mix cream cheese with parsley, lemon juice, and spices to make a green cream sauce. Season to taste. Set aside.
3. To make crepes, combine the flour, water, egg, egg white, and a couple of tablespoons of melted butter; beat to make a smooth dough.
4. Melt 1/2 tablespoon of butter in a skillet (8 to 10 inches crepe or sauté pan). Add 1/3 cup crepe batter and flip the pan to spread batter. Cook until bubbly and the edges begin to brown. Flip over and cook dinner briefly on the alternate side. Let cool on a plate. Repeat with the last butter and dough to make 4 crepes.
5. Spread crepes with cream cheese filling. Spread the asparagus lightly at the end of each crepe and roll tightly into rolls.
6. Wrap in aluminum foil and chill in the refrigerator for an hour. Cut chilled crepes into 3 or 4 pieces with a pointed knife before serving.

Nutritional value:
- Energy value: 190 Kcal
- Proteins: 5 g
- Carbohydrates: 12 g
- Fiber: 4 g
- Sugar: 4 g
- Sodium: 5 g
- Fat: 10g
  - *Of which:*
    - Saturated: 5 g
    - Monounsaturated: 7 g
    - Polyunsaturated: 4 g

Cholesterol: 111 mg

26. FESTIVE PINEAPPLE CHEESE BALL

Servings: 4
Ingredients:
24 ounces cream cheese
20 ounces crushed pineapple in a can
1/2 cup green bell pepper
1/4 teaspoon garlic powder

Instructions:
1. Place the softened cream cheese in a large mixing bowl.
2. Drain the pineapple well. Cut the bell pepper into small pieces.
3. To mix the ingredients, add to a bowl and stir well.
4. Shape the mixture into a ball. Wrap in wax paper and place in the refrigerator overnight.

Nutritional value:
- Energy value: 175 Kcal
- Proteins: 13 g
- Carbohydrates: 11 g
- Fiber: 3 g
- Sugar: 2 g
- Sodium: 3 g
- Fats: 11 g
  - *Of which:*
    - Saturated: 3 g
    - Monounsaturated: 5 g
    - Polyunsaturated: 2 g
- Cholesterol: 87 mg

27. FALAFEL

Servings: 2
Ingredients:
2 green onions
1 pound dried chickpeas
2 cups onion (white)
4 cloves of garlic
1/2 cup of parsley
1/4 cup of lemon juice
1 1/2 tablespoons flour
1/4 teaspoon of salt
1 teaspoon chopped coriander
1 teaspoon ground cumin
1 teaspoon cayenne pepper
1/4 teaspoon cayenne pepper

Instructions:
1. In a large pot, cover the chickpeas with water and soak overnight at room temperature.
2. Finely chop the white onion, as well as the chives, parsley, and garlic.
3. Chickpeas should be drained and rinsed. Combine green onion, white onion, parsley, garlic, lemon juice, flour, salt, coriander, cumin, black pepper, and cayenne pepper in a food processor.
4. Pulse until the mixture resembles a paste or coarse flour. (Be careful not to over-process.) Depending on the size of your food processor, you may need to make it in two batches. Remove the large chickpeas chunks and mix everything with a fork.
5. Let the falafel mixture cool for 2 hours.
6. Preheat the oven to 400 degrees Fahrenheit.
7. With cooking spray, line a muffin tin.
8. Scoop into 24 balls or roll mixture into balls and place directly into muffin tin. Preheat the oven to 350 degrees Fahrenheit and bake for 7 minutes. Remove the falafel from the oven, flip it over, and bake for another 7 minutes.

Nutritional value:
- Energy value: 210 Kcal
- Proteins: 7 g
- Carbohydrates: 16 g
- Fiber: 4 g
- Sugar: 5 g
- Sodium: 5 g
- Fat: 13 g
  - *Of which:*

- o Saturated: 5 g
- o Monounsaturated: 7 g
- o Polyunsaturated: 4 g
- Cholesterol: 107 mg

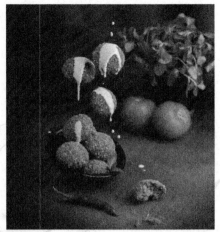

28. FRESH TOFU SPRING ROLLS

Servings: 4
Ingredients:

Romaine lettuce (12 sheets in total)
2 carrots, medium
1/2 red onion, medium
16 ounces firm tofu
1 tablespoon ground cumin
1/2 tablespoon garlic granules
1/4 teaspoon of salt
1/4 teaspoon of black pepper
1 tablespoon of extra virgin olive oil
12 rice wrappers (spring roll wrappers)

Instructions:

1. After washing and drying the lettuce, split each leaf lengthwise in half. Carrots should be julienned. Cut the onion into slices. Eliminate from the equation.
2. 6 cups water, bring to a boil and set aside to soak the rice wraps later.
3. The tofu should be drained and patted dry. It should be cut into 12 pieces, each about 4 inches long.
4. Season the tofu evenly with cumin, granulated garlic, sea salt, and black pepper on a plate.
5. With olive oil, heat a nonstick skillet. Place the seasoned side down in the skillet with the tofu strips. Season the other side and fry for 1 to 2 minutes, or until the bottom is slightly golden. Fry until the second side is lightly browned, then flip. To cool the tofu, place it on a plate.
6. Fill a wide, shallow container halfway with fresh water. In a bowl of hot water, soak a rice wrap. Place the wrap on a wide plate and place two lettuce halves in the center of the wrap until slightly fluffy. Over the lettuce, sprinkle 2 to 3 tablespoons of carrots and 1 to 2 tablespoons of sliced onion. On top of the vegetables, place a strip of cooled tofu.
7. Fold the sides in, then roll tightly from the bottom to the top. Using the remaining rice wrappers, veggies, and tofu strips, repeat the process.
8. Refrigerate and eat cold with a low sodium dressing of your choice.

Nutritional value:
- Energy value: 260 Kcal
- Proteins: 5 g
- Carbohydrates: 16 g
- Fiber: 4 g
- Sugar: 4 g
- Sodium: 5 g
- Fat: 18 g

- **Of which:**
  - o Saturated: 5 g
  - o Monounsaturated: 7 g
  - o Polyunsaturated: 4 g
- Cholesterol: 119 mg

29. AUTUMN WILD RICE

Servings: 4
Ingredients:

2 tablespoons raisins
Half a cup of short-cooked wild rice, uncooked
2 cups apples
34 cup carrots
1/4 cup celery
1/4 cup green bell pepper
1/4 teaspoon dried whole sage
1/4 teaspoon black pepper
1 half cups reduced-sodium chicken broth
3/4 cup converted rice, raw
1/4 cup clean lemon juice
1 sprig of clean sage (optionally available)

Instructions:

1. Combine raisins and 1/4 cup warm water; let stand 5 minutes. Drain and set aside.
2. Prepare quick-cooking wild rice following the Directions: on the package. Remove the pan from the heat and set it aside.
3. Chop the apples, celery, and bell pepper. Blend the carrot.
4. Coat a massive nonstick skillet with cooking spray; Place over medium-high heat until lukewarm. Add apple, celery, red pepper, and carrot; sauté until soft and crisp. Remove the pan from the heat and set it aside.
5. Combine 1 1/2 cup reduced-sodium poultry broth, sage, and pepper in a large saucepan; bring to a boil. Add the processed rice. Cover, reduce heat, and simmer 20 minutes or until rice is soft and liquid is absorbed.
6. Remove skillet from heat; Add reserved raisins, wild rice, apple sprinkle, and juice of 1 lemon. Cover and let stand 5 minutes.
7. Transfer to a serving bowl. Garnish with a sprig of sparkling sage, if you prefer.

Nutritional value:
- Energy value: 227 Kcal
- Proteins: 5 g
- Carbohydrates: 7 g
- Fiber: 5 g
- Sugar: 3 g
- Sodium: 2 g
- Fat: 9 g
  - **Of which:**
    - o Saturated: 7 g
    - o Monounsaturated: 1 g
    - o Polyunsaturated: 1 g
- Cholesterol: 100 mg

30. MAC-N-CHEESE WITH CAULIFLOWER AND BAKED BROCCOLI

Servings: 4
Ingredients:

12 ounces penne pasta, raw
2 cups cauliflower florets
2 cups broccoli florets
4 tablespoons unsalted butter
1/2 cup of onion
1 garlic clove
3 tablespoons all-purpose flour

2-1/2 cups Rice Dream® Classic Original rice drink
1/2 teaspoon black pepper
1/4 teaspoon of nutmeg
2 tablespoons spicy brown mustard
1 cup spicy white cheddar cheese, grated
1 cup of Swiss cheese, grated
1/2 piece of grated Parmesan cheese
1 cup panko-style breadcrumbs

Instructions:

1. Preheat the oven to 350 degrees Fahrenheit.
2. Bring the water to a boil. Add the pasta and cook over low heat for 2 min.
3. In a separate pot, steam broccoli and cauliflower florets for 5 minutes or until tender. Remove and reserve. Discard the liquid from the pot.
4. Finely chop the onion and garlic clove.
5. Using the identical pot, over medium heat, melt 3 tablespoons of butter and then load the onion and garlic. Sauté for 3–4 minutes, until smooth. Add the flour and beat for a minute. Stir in the rice drink and season with pepper and nutmeg. Stir until thickened, then stir in the highly spiced mustard.
6. Mix the 3 kinds of cheese together. Add 2/3 of the combined cheeses to the sauce and stir until the cheese is melted.
7. Drain the pasta. Add the cauliflower and broccoli then add the cheese sauce.
8. Spray a 9x12" baking pan with nonstick cooking spray and pour in the batter. Top with the remaining combination of cheeses.
9. Place the baking sheet inside the oven on the pinnacle of a baking sheet to catch the bubbles. After half an hour of baking, the temperature rises to 400 degrees Fahrenheit. Sauté the last tablespoon of butter with 1 cup of panko breadcrumbs and add to the top of the casserole. Cook for an additional 8 to 10 minutes until the breadcrumbs are golden brown.

Nutritional value:

- Energy value: 186 Kcal
- Proteins: 7 g
- Carbohydrates: 12 g
- Fiber: 9 g
- Sugar: 2 g
- Sodium: 4 g
- Fats: 15 g
  Of which:
  - Saturated: 5 g
  - Monounsaturated: 4 g
  - Polyunsaturated: 5 g

Cholesterol: 137 mg

FISH

31. BAKED SHRIMP ROLLS

Servings: 4
Ingredients:

2 quarts of Napa Valley cabbage
1/2 cup carrots
1/4 cup of green onions
2 teaspoons coriander chopped
1 teaspoon ginger root
1 1/2 cups shrimp, raw
1 tablespoon hoisin sauce
1 teaspoon sugar (brown)
1 teaspoon garlic powder
1/4 teaspoon red chili flakes (optional)
3 tablespoons water
12 7x7" egg roll wrappers

Instructions:

1. Preheat the oven to 400 degrees Fahrenheit. If the egg roll wrappers are frozen, place them to thaw.
2. Cabbage and carrots must be finely chopped. The onions should be thinly sliced and the cilantro should be minced. The ginger root must be grated.
3. Shrimp should be cleaned and finely chopped.
4. In a preheated nonstick skillet, combine the cabbage, carrots, shrimp, and green onions.
5. Cook, stirring regularly, over medium heat until shrimp are pink and vegetables are translucent and soft (about 8 minutes).
6. Combine cilantro, hoisin sauce, brown sugar, garlic powder, ginger, and red chili flakes in a large mixing bowl.
7. Mix well to make sure the spices are evenly distributed.
8. Cook for another 2 minutes, then remove from heat and drain excess liquid.
9. Drizzle a baking sheet with canola oil and set aside while the shrimp vegetable mixture cools.
10. Fill spring roll wrappers as follows on a cutting board (or another clean surface): Place a heaping tablespoon of cooked batter diagonally on each wrapper, about a third of the way from the top, but not directly in the middle. Fold two opposite edges of the wrap over the filling, then roll the shorter side first, then the longer side, until the roll is complete.
11. Place the folded edge down on a baking sheet after dipping a finger in water and rubbing along the edge of the entire roll to close it.
12. Drizzle canola oil on each filled spring roll.
13. Preheat oven to 350 degrees Fahrenheit and bake for 20 minutes, turning after 10 minutes. The muffins should be lightly browned and crisp on the outside.

Nutritional value:		
• Energy value: 227 Kcal		
• Proteins: 5 g		
• Carbohydrates: 7 g		
• Fiber: 5 g		
• Sugar: 3 g		
• Sodium: 2 g		
• Fat: 9 g		
Of which:		
	o Saturated: 7 g	
	o Monounsaturated: 1 g	
	o Polyunsaturated: 1 g	
• Cholesterol: 100 mg		

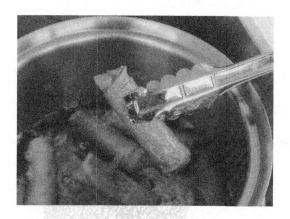

32. CRAB STUFFED CELERY LOGS

Servings: 2
Ingredients:

4 ribs of celery (medium 8-inch)
1 tablespoon red onion
1/4 cup crab meat
2 tablespoons mayonnaise
1/4 teaspoon of lemon juice
1/4 teaspoon paprika

Instructions:

1. Trim the ends of the celery ribs. Drain the crab meat and shred it. Finely chop the onion.
2. Combine the crabmeat, onion, mayo, and lemon juice in a small bowl.
3. 1 tablespoon of the crab mixture should be stuffed into each celery bone.
4. Each rib of celery should be cut into three sections.
5. Until serving, sprinkle paprika over the pieces of celery stuffed with crab.

Nutritional value:		
• Energy value: 186 Kcal		
• Proteins: 7 g		
• Carbohydrates: 12 g		
• Fiber: 9 g		
• Sugar: 2 g		
• Sodium: 4 g		
• Fats: 15 g		
Of which:		
	o Saturated: 5 g	
	o Monounsaturated: 4 g	
	o Polyunsaturated: 5 g	
Cholesterol: 137 mg		

33. BAGEL WITH EGG AND SALMON

Servings: 2
Ingredients:

1/2 bagel
1 tablespoon cream cheese
1 tablespoon chives
1/2 teaspoon sparkling dill
2 clean basil leaves
1 tomato slice
4 servings of arugula
1 large egg
1 ounce of cooked salmon

Instructions:

1. Cut the bagel in half and toast half in a toaster or oven.
2. Chop the chives, dill, and basil leaves. Mix with the cream cheese.
3. Spread cream cheese combo on 1/2 toasted bagel, then garnish with arugula and a tomato wedge.
4. Heat a frying pan, spray with nonstick spray and stir the egg.
5. Reheat the salmon in the skillet at the same time the egg cooks.
6. Place the egg and salmon on the pinnacle of the tomato slice. Enjoy!

Nutritional value:

- Energy value: 153 Kcal
- Proteins: 7 g
- Carbohydrates: 16 g
- Fiber: 7 g
- Sugar: 5 g
- Sodium: 2 g
- Fats: 13 g
  Of which:
  - Saturated: 4 g
  - Monounsaturated: 6 g
  - Polyunsaturated: 2 g

Cholesterol: 115 mg

MEATS

34. CHICKEN CUBES

Servings: 2
Ingredients:

3/4 pound chicken breasts, with the skin and bones removed
3 tablespoons cream cheese
1 tablespoon unsalted butter
1/2 cup of broccoli florets
1 package of Pillsbury® Original Crescent Rolls

Instructions:

1. Preheat the oven to 350 degrees Fahrenheit. Place the cream cheese to melt. Melt butter.
2. Cook, drain, and chop the broccoli.
3. Boil the poultry breasts until they are cooked; drain, discard the skin and bones and cut them into portions.
4. Mix together the chicken, softened cream cheese, melted butter, and broccoli.
5. Open the crescent rolls and form a rectangle with 2 rolls. Pinch the seam to seal and stretch the rectangle.
6. Place 1/4 of the chicken aggregate in the center. Fold the edges to make a rotation. Press edges to seal.
7. Bake 25 to 30 minutes or until muffins are golden brown.

> **Nutritional value:**
> - Energy value: 175 Kcal
> - Proteins: 13 g
> - Carbohydrates: 11 g
> - Fiber: 3 g
> - Sugar: 2 g
> - Sodium: 3 g
> - Fats: 11 g
>   ***Of which:***
>   - Saturated: 3 g
>   - Monounsaturated: 5 g
>   - Polyunsaturated: 2 g
> - Cholesterol: 87 mg

35. BARBECUED MEATBALLS

Servings: 4
Ingredients:

1 pound onion
3 pounds beef (ground)
2 chickens, large
1/2 cup unenriched rice milk
1 cup of raw oatmeal
1 tablespoon dried thyme
1 teaspoon dried oregano
1/2 teaspoon of pepper
1 liter of barbecue sauce
1/3 cup liquid

Instructions:

1. Preheat the oven to 375 degrees Fahrenheit.
2. The onion should be diced and the eggs should be beaten.
3. In a large bowl, combine all ingredients (except barbecue sauce and water) and stir to combine.
4. Place on a baking sheet and roll into 1" balls.
5. Cook 10–15 minutes or until meatballs are cooked through.
6. In a warming dish or crock pot over low heat, combine the barbecue sauce and wine. Add the meatballs. Cover and reserve until ready to serve.

> **Nutritional value:**
> - Energy value: 260 Kcal
> - Proteins: 5 g
> - Carbohydrates: 16 g
> - Fiber: 4 g
> - Sugar: 4 g
> - Sodium: 5 g
> - Fat: 18 g
>   ***Of which:***
>   - Saturated: 5 g
>   - Monounsaturated: 7 g
>   - Polyunsaturated: 4 g
>
> Cholesterol: 119 mg

36. MEAT BURRITOS

Servings: 2
Ingredients:

1/4 cup onion
1/4 cup green bell pepper
1 pound lean ground beef
1 tablespoon tomato puree (low sodium)
1/4 teaspoon black pepper
1 tablespoon ground cumin
Flour tortillas, burrito size

Instructions:

1. The green pepper and onion should be chopped.
2. Brown the ground beef in a medium skillet and drain.
3. Spray skillet with nonstick cooking spray, then add onion and green bell pepper, cook 3 to 5 minutes, until vegetables are tender.
4. To the onion/bell pepper mixture, add the meat, tomato puree, black pepper, and cumin, and stir well. Cook for 3 to 5 minutes over low heat.
5. Fill the tortillas halfway with the meat mixture. To prevent the mixture from falling off, roll the tortilla into a burrito shape, folding both ends first.

> **Nutritional value:**
> - Energy value: 186 Kcal
> - Proteins: 7 g
> - Carbohydrates: 12 g
> - Fiber: 9 g
> - Sugar: 2 g
> - Sodium: 4 g
> - Fats: 15 g
>   ***Of which:***
>   - Saturated: 5 g
>   - Monounsaturated: 4 g
>   - Polyunsaturated: 5 g
> - Cholesterol: 137 mg

37. BUFFALO WINGS

Servings: 2
Ingredients:

8 tablespoons butter (unsalted)
1/3 cup Tabasco® chili sauce
1/4 cup red pepper sauce (roasted)
1/4 cup tomato sauce (low sodium)
1 tablespoon of extra virgin olive oil
1/4 teaspoon garlic powder
1/2 teaspoon Italian seasoning mix (dry)
2 teaspoons hot sauce

Instructions:

1. Preheat the oven to 400 degrees Fahrenheit.
2. In a saucepan, melt the butter.
3. Stir to combine the hot sauce, red pepper sauce, tomato sauce, olive oil, garlic powder, and Italian seasonings. Turn off the heat in the skillet.
4. In a baking dish, place the chicken wings.
5. Bake for 30 to 35 minutes after pouring the sauce over the wings. Check if something has finished.
6. Serve wings immediately or keep warm on a covered plate or crock pot until ready to eat.

Nutritional value:
- Energy value: 153 Kcal
- Proteins: 7 g
- Carbohydrates: 16 g
- Fiber: 7 g
- Sugar: 5 g
- Sodium: 2 g
- Fats: 13 g
    Of which:
    - Saturated: 4 g
    - Monounsaturated: 6 g
    - Polyunsaturated: 2 g

Cholesterol: 115 mg

38. AUTHENTIC BEEF TACOS

Servings: 4
Ingredients:

1 pound skirt or flank steak (skirt)
2 teaspoons Mrs. Dash® Lemon Pepper Seasoning Blend
3 limes
2 teaspoons garlic powder
1 tablespoon of coriander
1 tablespoon of onion
3 garlic cloves
2 teaspoons of extra virgin olive oil
8 flour tortillas (6")
1/2 cup of fresh cheese from Mexico

Instructions:
1. For 30 minutes to overnight, marinate the steak on a flat plate with the juice of two lemons, lemon pepper, and garlic powder.
2. The coriander should be finely chopped and the onion and garlic should be diced. To make the sauce, combine the cilantro, onion, garlic, and 1 lime juice. Cover and store in the refrigerator.
3. 2 tablespoons oil, heated over medium-high heat. Finely chop the steak and cook until cooked through, about 3 minutes per side.
4. Preheat the oven to 350 degrees Fahrenheit.
5. Fill the flour tortilla with an equal amount of cooked steak, about 1-1 / 2 ounces.
6. Crumbled 1 tablespoon of fresh cheese on top of each taco.
7. Wrap each taco in aluminum foil and bake for 5 to 8 minutes, or until the tortillas are soft.
8. Take the dish out of the oven. Enjoy your tacos with salsa on top!

Nutritional value:
- Energy value: 192 Kcal
- Proteins: 19 g
- Carbohydrates: 15 g
- Fiber: 7 g
- Sugar: 3 g
- Sodium: 3 g
- Fats: 10 g
    Of which:
    - Saturated: 5 g
    - Monounsaturated: 3 g
    - Polyunsaturated: 1 g

Cholesterol: 127 mg

39. BROCCOLI AND BEEF STIR FRY

Servings: 4
Ingredients:

2 cloves of garlic
1 Roma tomato, medium
8 ounces uncooked lean beef tenderloin
12 ounces broccoli, frozen vegetable mix in a stir fry
2 tablespoons peanut butter
1/4 cup chicken broth (low sodium)
1 tablespoon of cornstarch
2 tablespoons soy sauce (low sodium)
2 cups of rice (cooked)

Instructions:
1. Chop the Roma tomato and garlic cloves. The meat should be cut into thin strips.
2. Thaw frozen stir fry vegetable mix in microwave on defrost setting for 3–4 minutes.
3. Heat the oil in a frying pan or wok and fry the garlic until fragrant. Sauté the vegetable mixture for about 5 minutes or until cooked. Remove the pan from the heat and set it aside.
4. Add the meat to the same plate. Cook for about 7 minutes, or until the meat is cooked to your liking.
5. In a mixing plate, combine the chicken broth, cornstarch, and soy sauce.
6. In the same skillet as the meat, add the cooked vegetables, sauce, and tomato. Cook, stirring constantly until sauce thickens.
7. 1/2 cup of brown rice should be served with this dish.

Nutritional value:
- Energy value: 160 Kcal
- Proteins: 5 g
- Carbohydrates: 16 g
- Fiber: 4 g
- Sugar: 4 g
- Sodium: 5 g
- Fat: 18 g
    Of which:
    - Saturated: 5 g
    - Monounsaturated: 7 g
    - Polyunsaturated: 4 g

Cholesterol: 109 mg

40. APPLE SPICED PORK CHOPS

Servings: 4
Ingredients:

2 tablespoons butter
1 pound pork chops
1/4 cup of brown sugar
1/4 teaspoon salt
1/5 teaspoon of pepper
1/5 teaspoon of nutmeg
1/5 teaspoon of cinnamon
2 apples, medium pie

Instructions:
1. Preheat the broiler in the oven.
2. Apples should be peeled, cored, and sliced.
3. Grill the pork chops for 4 to 5 minutes per side in the oven.
4. Melt the butter in a skillet and add brown sugar, salt, pepper, nutmeg, cinnamon, and apples while the pork chops cook.
5. Cook, covered, until apples are tender and sauce thickens.
6. Serve the sauce over the fried cutlets.

Nutritional value:
- Energy value: 186 Kcal
- Proteins: 7 g
- Carbohydrates: 12 g

- Fiber: 9 g
- Sugar: 2 g
- Sodium: 4 g
- Fats: 15 g
  - *Of which:*
    - o Saturated: 5 g
    - o Monounsaturated: 4 g
    - o Polyunsaturated: 5 g
- Cholesterol: 137 mg

41. CHICKEN ENCHILADAS

Servings: 4

Ingredients:

2 tablespoons canola oil
12 corn tortillas, 6" long
3 cups of chicken breast, cooked and shredded
2/3 cup onion, finely chopped
1/2 cup light sour cream
1/2 cup enchilada sauce

Instructions:

1. Preheat the oven to 375 degrees Fahrenheit.
2. Heat the oil in a skillet.
3. Quickly dip each tortilla in a skillet to soften, then discard on a plate.
4. In the center of each tortilla, 1/4 cup crumbled chicken, 1 tablespoon onion, and 2 teaspoons sour cream.
5. Roll and surround each enchilada in a baking dish.
6. Top with 1–1/2 cups enchilada sauce.
7. Place the baking dish in the oven and heat for 20 to 30 minutes or until hot.

Nutritional value:
- Energy value: 260 Kcal
- Proteins: 5 g
- Carbohydrates: 16 g
- Fiber: 4 g
- Sugar: 4 g
- Sodium: 5 g
- Fat: 18 g
  - *Of which:*
    - o Saturated: 5 g
    - o Monounsaturated: 7 g
    - o Polyunsaturated: 4 g
- Cholesterol: 119 mg

42. ROAST CHICKEN, ASPARAGUS, AND CORN

Servings: 2

Ingredients:

8 ounces boneless skinless chicken breast (1 large breast or 2 medium breasts)
2 tablespoons olive oil
1/2 teaspoon ground black pepper
1/2 teaspoon of herb and spice mix (cumin, paprika, chili powder)
1/4 teaspoon pepper flakes
10 asparagus
1 clean corncob (Colorado corn, if you have one)
1/2 lemon
1 tablespoon clean chives

Instructions:

1. Season the chicken with a tablespoon of olive oil, ground black pepper, herb and spice mix, and crushed red pepper flakes. Add the chicken to the hot spot on the grill, seasoned side down. Roast for 12 minutes.
2. While the chicken is cooking, reduce the asparagus and grill area. Season with black pepper and drizzle with 2 teaspoons of olive oil. Grill the asparagus for 5 to 7 minutes.
3. Cut the corn on the cob in half and drizzle with 1 teaspoon of olive oil. Grill the corn for 3–4 minutes, until slightly charred.

After removing the corn from the grill, add a splash of lemon juice and chopped chives.

4. Squeeze the lemon over the bird and the asparagus to taste.

Nutritional value:
- Energy value: 153 Kcal
- Proteins: 7 g
- Carbohydrates: 16 g
- Fiber: 7 g
- Sugar: 5 g
- Sodium: 2 g
- Fats: 13 g
  - *Of which:*
    - o Saturated: 4 g
    - o Monounsaturated: 6 g
    - o Polyunsaturated: 2 g

Cholesterol: 115 mg

43. CHORIZO AND EGG OMELET

Servings: 1

Ingredients:

1/4 cup of chorizo
1 large egg
2 corn tortillas, 6 inches long

Instructions:

1. Cook 1/4 cup chorizo in a skillet on the stove, cutting the meat into large crumbs with a spatula.
2. Drain excess fat and water, if desired. Once the meat is cooked through, add 1 egg, stirring to combine while the egg cooks.
3. Serve with 2 corn tortillas.

Nutritional value:
- Energy value: 186 Kcal
- Proteins: 7 g
- Carbohydrates: 12 g
- Fiber: 9 g
- Sugar: 2 g
- Sodium: 4 g
- Fats: 15 g
  - *Of which:*
    - o Saturated: 5 g
    - o Monounsaturated: 4 g
    - o Polyunsaturated: 5 g
- Cholesterol: 137 mg

44. CHICKEN PASTA WITH BRUSSELS SPROUTS

Servings: 2

Ingredients:

1/2 cup of onions
1/2 cup red bell pepper
1/2 cup fresh or frozen Brussels sprouts
1 1/2 cups cooked whole wheat rotini pasta
1 tablespoon butter
1 tablespoon canola oil
1 tablespoon low sodium soy sauce
1-1/2 cups cooked poultry, cubed

Instructions:

1. Chop the onions and red peppers.
2. Cut off the ends of the Brussels sprouts and boil or steam until tender.
3. Cook pasta according to the instructions on the package, but omit salt.
4. While pasta is cooking, drain Brussels sprouts and set them aside.
5. Heat the butter and oil and sauté the onions in a skillet.

6. Add the red bell peppers and Brussels sprouts, stirring until brown around the edges.
7. Add the soy sauce and cook until the pasta is done.
8. Microwave the poultry if you like.
9. Combine pasta, poultry, and cooked vegetables in a bowl.
10. Serve at once while hot.

Nutritional value:
- Energy value: 192 Kcal
- Proteins: 19 g
- Carbohydrates: 15 g
- Fiber: 7 g
- Sugar: 3 g
- Sodium: 3 g
- Fats: 10 g
  Of which:
  - Saturated: 5 g
  - Monounsaturated: 3 g
  - Polyunsaturated: 1 g
- Cholesterol: 127 mg

45. CHICKEN WITH BLUEBERRIES

Servings: 4
Ingredients:

1 tablespoon of olive oil
1/4 cup onion
2 pounds boneless, skinless bird breasts
1/4 cup ketchup
1 teaspoon dry mustard
16 ounces canned cranberry sauce
1/4 cup brown sugar
1 tablespoon apple cider vinegar

Instructions:
1. Chop the onion.
2. Preheat the oil in a large skillet. Add the onion and sauté until clean.
3. Add the bird and cook for 3 to 4 minutes on each facet.
4. In a medium bowl, combine ketchup, dry mustard, cranberry sauce, packed brown sugar, and vinegar. Stir until combined and pour into a skillet.
5. Cover and cook on medium heat for 15 to 20 minutes.

Nutritional value:
- Energy value: 175 Kcal
- Proteins: 13 g
- Carbohydrates: 11 g
- Fiber: 3 g
- Sugar: 2 g
- Sodium: 3 g
- Fats: 11 g
  Of which:
  - Saturated: 3 g
  - Monounsaturated: 5 g
  - Polyunsaturated: 2 g

Cholesterol: 87 mg

46. CROCK-POT ORIENTAL CHICKEN

Servings: 3
Ingredients:

2 medium carrots
2 onions
4 ribs of celery
1 garlic clove
8 ounces canned bamboo shoots
8 ounces canned water chestnuts
2 tablespoons vegetable oil
6 boneless skinless chicken breasts
1 cup low sodium chicken broth
1 tablespoon of brown sugar

1/4 cup low sodium soy sauce
1/4 teaspoon crushed pink pepper flakes
1/4 cup cornstarch
1/3 cup of water
3 cups of cooked white rice

Instructions:
1. Cut the carrots, chives, and sliced celery. Crush the garlic. Rinse and slice the bamboo shoots and water chestnuts.
2. Heat the oil in a frying pan and fry all the sides.
3. Transfer the bird to a crock pot.
4. Add all the ingredients except the cornstarch and water. Cook dinner on low heat setting for 6 to 8 hours.
5. Mix cornstarch and water, stirring until smooth, then mix with Crock-Pot liquid. Place the lid of the slow cooker ajar to allow steam to escape. Cook over high heat until thickened, about 15 minutes.
6. Serve chicken and vegetables over rice.

Nutritional value:
- Energy value: 113 Kcal
- Proteins: 13 g
- Carbohydrates: 8 g
- Fiber: 9 g
- Sugar: 4 g
- Sodium: 4 g
- Fats: 10 g
  Of which:
  - Saturated: 2 g
  - Monounsaturated: 2 g
  - Polyunsaturated: 4 g
- Cholesterol: 127 mg

47. CHICKEN VERONIQUE

Servings: 2
Ingredients:

2 boneless skinless chicken breasts (4 ounces each)
2 butter spoons
1/2 shallot
1 teaspoon cornstarch
2 tablespoons dry white wine
2 tablespoons low sodium chicken broth
1/2 cup of seedless grapes
1 teaspoon dried tarragon
1/4 cup cream

Instructions:
1. In an 8-inch skillet, heat butter and brown poultry breasts on both sides until golden brown. Remove to a plate.
2. Finely chop the shallot and sauté until soft.
3. In a small bowl, whisk the cornstarch with the wine and broth. Pour into the pan, stir, and then turn up the chicken breasts. Cover and simmer for 5 to 6 minutes.
4. While the chicken simmers, cut the grapes in half.
5. Remove the chicken from the skillet and cover to keep warm. Add the cream and tarragon to the skillet and bring to a boil. Add the grapes to the sauce and cook dinner until hot.
6. Place each poultry breast on a plate and pour the sauce and grapes over the top.

Nutritional value:
- Energy value: 186 Kcal
- Proteins: 7 g
- Carbohydrates: 12 g
- Fiber: 9 g
- Sugar: 2 g
- Sodium: 4 g
- Fats: 15 g
  Of which:
  - Saturated: 5 g
  - Monounsaturated: 4 g
  - Polyunsaturated: 5 g

Cholesterol: 137 mg

48. GLAZED CORNISH HEN FOR TWO

Servings: 1
Ingredients:

1-1/4 pound Cornish hen
3 tablespoons of butter
2 tablespoons apricot jam
1 teaspoon Dijon mustard
1 teaspoon Worcestershire sauce

Instructions:

1. Preheat the oven to 375 degrees Fahrenheit. In a small saucepan, melt the butter.
2. Remove and discard the giblets from the hollow space of the thawed Cornish hen. Rinse and pat dry. Rub the skin and internal hollows with a tablespoon of melted butter. Place the chicken in the oven and bake for 20 minutes.
3. Add jam, mustard, and Worcestershire sauce to last melted butter; heat and stir until just combined.
4. After baking for 20 minutes, brush the chicken with the apricot glaze. Bake 20 to 30 more minutes, basting with frosting every 10 minutes. Remove from oven when internal temperature reaches 165 degrees Fahrenheit.
5. Let the bird rest for 10 minutes and then cut it in half and place it on serving plates. Heat final frosting to a boil then pour in each half before serving.

Nutritional value:
- Energy value: 260 Kcal
- Proteins: 5 g
- Carbohydrates: 16 g
- Fiber: 4 g
- Sugar: 4 g
- Sodium: 5 g
- Fat: 18 g
  Of which:
  - Saturated: 5 g
  - Monounsaturated: 7 g
  - Polyunsaturated: 4 g
- Cholesterol: 119 mg

49. LOW PROTEIN BEEF TIBBS

Servings: 1
Ingredients:

1 medium onion
1 medium tomato
1 green bell pepper, medium
8 ounces lean beef stew
2 tablespoons olive oil
1/4 teaspoon salt
1/5 teaspoon of black pepper

Instructions:

1. The onion must be cut into thin slices. The tomato and bell pepper should be chopped. The meat should be cut into small cubes.
2. In a frying pan, sauté the onion and oil until the onion is slightly orange.
3. Add the meat and tomatoes.
4. Add bell pepper or jalapeño after partially cooked.
5. Cook until meat is tender, about 15 more minutes.
6. Season with salt and pepper before serving.

Nutritional value:
- Energy value: 186 Kcal
- Proteins: 7 g
- Carbohydrates: 12 g
- Fiber: 9 g
- Sugar: 2 g
- Sodium: 4 g
- Fats: 15 g

Of which:
- Saturated: 5 g
- Monounsaturated: 4 g
- Polyunsaturated: 5 g
- Cholesterol: 137 mg

50. BREWERY BURGER

Servings: 4
Ingredients:

3 tablespoons rice milk
5 soda crackers (unsalted)
1 large egg
1 teaspoon herb seasoning mix (unsalted)
1 pound 85 percent lean ground beef

Instructions:

1. In a bowl, crush the soda crackers and mix them with the milk. Let stand until the cookies are soft.
2. In a separate bowl, beat the egg and add it to the cookie mix. Mix the herb mixture well, breaking up the cookies as needed. Mix the ground beef well.
3. Create 4 equal-sized patties with the ground beef mixture.
4. Grill over medium heat until the internal temperature reaches at least 160 degrees Fahrenheit.
5. Serve on a bun with your favorite toppings or as a patty with your choice of vegetables and starch.

Nutritional value:
- Energy value: 227 Kcal
- Proteins: 5 g
- Carbohydrates: 7 g
- Fiber: 5 g
- Sugar: 3 g
- Sodium: 2 g
- Fat: 9 g
  Of which:
  - Saturated: 7 g
  - Monounsaturated: 1 g
  - Polyunsaturated: 1 g
- Cholesterol: 100 mg

51. CHICKEN NUGGETS WITH MUSTARD HONEY SAUCE

Servings: 3
Ingredients:

1 tablespoon mustard (yellow)
1/2 cup mayonnaise
2 teaspoons Worcestershire sauce
1/3 cup honey
1 large egg
1/4 cup of milk with a fat content of 1%
3 quarts corn flakes
1 pound boneless chicken breast

Instructions:

1. In a small bowl, combine the mustard, mayonnaise, honey, and Worcestershire sauce. Chill the sauce until the nuggets are set, then use as a dipping sauce.
2. Preheat the oven to 400 degrees Fahrenheit.
3. Chicken breast should be cut into 36 bite-size pieces.
4. The cornflakes should be crushed and poured into a large zip-lock bag.
5. In a small bowl, combine the beaten egg and milk. After dipping the chicken parts into the egg mixture, shake them in a zip-lock bag to coat with corn flake crumbs.
6. Bake nuggets for 15 minutes or until baked on a baking sheet coated with nonstick cooking spray.

Nutritional value:
- Energy value: 175 Kcal
- Proteins: 13 g
- Carbohydrates: 11 g
- Fiber: 3 g
- Sugar: 2 g
- Sodium: 3 g
- Fats: 11 g
  Of which:
  - Saturated: 3 g
  - Monounsaturated: 5 g
  - Polyunsaturated: 2 g
- Cholesterol: 87 mg

52. LOW PROTEIN BURGER BREWERY

Servings: 4
Ingredients:

3 tablespoons rice milk
7 unsalted soda crackers
1 large egg
1 teaspoon herb seasoning mix (unsalted)
1 pound 85 percent lean ground beef

Instructions:

1. In a bowl, combine milk and crushed cookies; reserve until cookies are soft.
2. Mix in beaten egg and herb seasoning mixture, breaking cookies as desired. Mix the ground beef well.
3. Create 6 patties of equal size with the mixture.
4. Roast over medium heat until finished to your liking.

Nutritional value:
- Energy value: 186 Kcal
- Proteins: 7 g
- Carbohydrates: 12 g
- Fiber: 9 g
- Sugar: 2 g
- Sodium: 4 g
- Fats: 15 g
  Of which:
  - Saturated: 5 g
  - Monounsaturated: 4 g
  - Polyunsaturated: 5 g
- Cholesterol: 137 mg

53. CHICKEN, PEPPER, AND BACON WRAPS

Servings: 4
Ingredients:

1 medium onion
12 strips of bacon
12 jalapeno peppers, fresh
12 banana peppers, fresh
2 ounces boneless, skinless chicken breasts
24 toothpicks, no color tint

Instructions:

1. With a sharp knife, cut the onion into chunks. The bacon can be cut in half.
2. Spray the grill grate with a high-heat nonstick cooking spray. Preheat an outdoor grill or an indoor grill.
3. Remove the seeds from the inside of the peppers before cooking. To break up the pepper, cut it along one side.
4. Cut the chicken into 24 pieces, each large enough to fit inside the peppers.
5. Fill each pepper with a piece of chicken. It's okay if some of the chicken escapes the pepper.

6. To coat the chicken, place a slice of onion on top.
7. Wrap the bacon around the tomato, chicken, and onion, and secure with toothpicks. For added safety, use several toothpicks inserted in different directions.
8. Place on the grill to cook.
9. Cook 10–15 minutes or until bacon is crisp. To prevent the flames from burning the bacon while the fat drips, flip and turn frequently.

Nutritional value:
- Energy value: 153 Kcal
- Proteins: 7 g
- Carbohydrates: 16 g
- Fiber: 7 g
- Sugar: 5 g
- Sodium: 2 g
- Fats: 13 g
  Of which:
  - Saturated: 4 g
  - Monounsaturated: 6 g
  - Polyunsaturated: 2 g
- Cholesterol: 115 mg

54. PORK CHOPS WITH APPLE AND STUFFING

Servings: 3
Ingredients:

Stove Top® Chicken Stuffing Mix
2 tablespoons margarine (without salt)
1 jar or can (20 ounces) Apple Pie Filling
6 pork loin chops (boneless)

Instructions:

1. Preheat the oven to 350 Fahrenheit degrees.
2. Coat a 9x13" baking pan with cooking spray.
3. Set the filling mixture, water, and margarine aside in a mixing bowl according to the package directions.
4. Cover the bottom of the pan with apple pie filling.
5. Place the pork chops on top of the apple pie filling.
6. Fill the pork chops with stuffing.
7. Bake for 30 minutes, covered with foil.
8. Remove the foil and bake for another 10 minutes.

Nutritional value:
- Energy value: 260 Kcal
- Proteins: 5 g
- Carbohydrates: 16 g
- Fiber: 4 g
- Sugar: 4 g
- Sodium: 5 g
- Fat: 18 g
  Of which:
  - Saturated: 5 g
  - Monounsaturated: 7 g
  - Polyunsaturated: 4 g
- Cholesterol: 119 mg

55. APPLE SPICED PORK CHOPS

Servings: 4
Ingredients:

1 pound pork chops
1/4 cup brown sugar
2 butter spoons
1/4 teaspoon of salt
1/4 teaspoon of pepper
1/4 teaspoon of nutmeg
1/4 teaspoon of cinnamon
2 apples, medium pie

Instructions:

1. Preheat the broiler in the oven.
2. Apples should be peeled, cored, and sliced.
3. Grill the pork chops for 4 to 5 minutes per side in the oven.
4. Melt the butter in a skillet and add brown sugar, salt, pepper, nutmeg, cinnamon, and apples while the pork chops cook.
5. Cook, covered until apples are tender and sauce thickens.
6. Serve the sauce over the cooked chops.

Nutritional value:
- Energy value: 186 Kcal
- Proteins: 7 g
- Carbohydrates: 12 g
- Fiber: 9 g
- Sugar: 2 g
- Sodium: 4 g
- Fats: 15 g
  Of which:
    o Saturated: 5 g
    o Monounsaturated: 4 g
    o Polyunsaturated: 5 g
- Cholesterol: 137 mg

56. BAKED PORK CHOPS

Servings: 3
Ingredients:

1/2 cup all-purpose flour
1 large egg
1 cup of water
1/3 cup corn flake crumbs
6 3-1/2-ounce pork chops, cut medium
2 tablespoons margarine (unsalted)
1 teaspoon paprika
1/4 teaspoon salt
6 peach halves in juice, canned

Instructions:

1. Preheat the oven to 350 degrees Fahrenheit.
2. In a shallow pan or plate, add the flour and salt.
3. On a small plate, beat the egg and water mixture. In a shallow dish, spread the corn flake crumbs.
4. To coat the pork chops, dredge them in flour. Dredge each cutlet in corn flake crumbs after dipping into the egg mixture.
5. Place the chops on a baking sheet that has been lightly sprayed with nonstick cooking spray. Drizzle melted margarine on top.
6. Refrigerate the chops for at least 1 hour after sprinkling them with paprika and salt.
7. Preheat the oven to 400 degrees Fahrenheit and bake the pork chops for 40 minutes or until done.
8. Grill the drained peach halves in a skillet and serve with half a peach on top of each pork chop.

Nutritional value:
- Energy value: 227 Kcal
- Proteins: 5 g
- Carbohydrates: 7 g
- Fiber: 5 g
- Sugar: 3 g
- Sodium: 2 g
- Fat: 9 g
  Of which:
    o Saturated: 7 g
    o Monounsaturated: 1 g
    o Polyunsaturated: 1 g
Cholesterol: 100 mg

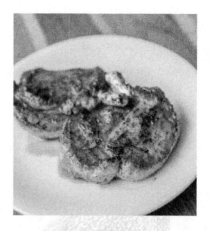

57. BRAISED BEEF RIBS

Servings: 4
Ingredients:

1 pound carrots
1 cup of celery
1 pound onion
2 1/2 pounds boneless short ribs
2 teaspoons all-purpose flour plus 1/2 cup all-purpose flour
1/5 teaspoon of black pepper
A fraction of a cup of canola oil
2 cups beef broth (low sodium)

Instructions:

1. Preheat the oven to 350 degrees Fahrenheit.
2. The carrot, celery, and onion should be chopped.
3. The ribs must be free of fat. Combine 1/2 cup of the flour and pepper on a mixing plate. To coat the ribs, roll them in flour.
4. In a skillet, heat 1–1/2 tablespoons of oil and brown the ribs on all sides.
5. Place the ribs in a roasting pan and grill for 45 minutes, uncovered. Remove excess fat carefully.
6. In a large pot, heat 1/2 tablespoon of the oil and sauté the chopped vegetables until tender.
7. Add the beef broth and the roast ribs. Cook over low heat for 2 hours, or until the ribs are tender.
8. Brown 2 tablespoons of flour in 1 tablespoon of oil to create a sauce. Add 1 cup of the meat liquid and stir until thickened over medium heat. With each serving of ribs, add 2 tablespoons of sauce.

Nutritional value:
- Energy value: 192 Kcal
- Proteins: 19 g
- Carbohydrates: 15 g
- Fiber: 7 g
- Sugar: 3 g
- Sodium: 3 g
- Fats: 10 g
  Of which:
    o Saturated: 5 g
    o Monounsaturated: 3 g
    o Polyunsaturated: 1 g
- Cholesterol: 127 mg

58. EASY CHICKEN AND PASTA DINNER

Servings: 4
Ingredients:

1 tablespoon of olive oil
1/2 cup red bell pepper, sliced
1 cup zucchini sliced

49

2 cups cooked pasta, any shape
5 ounces cooked poultry breast
3 tablespoons low sodium Italian dressing

Instructions:

1. In a nonstick skillet, heat the olive oil and sauté the zucchini and bell peppers until crisp-tender. Remove to a plate.
2. Cut the birds into strips.
3. Microwave cooked pasta and chicken strips on separate plates.
4. Toss the pasta with the Italian dressing. Top with strips of poultry and sautéed vegetables.

Nutritional value:
- Energy value: 153 Kcal
- Proteins: 7 g
- Carbohydrates: 16 g
- Fiber: 7 g
- Sugar: 5 g
- Sodium: 2 g
- Fats: 13 g
  Of which:
    - Saturated: 4 g
    - Monounsaturated: 6 g
    - Polyunsaturated: 2 g

Cholesterol: 115 mg

59. CHICKEN AND RICE CASSEROLE

Servings: 4

Ingredients:

1 cup of bell pepper
1/2 cup of onion
2 tablespoons olive oil
2 spoons of butter
1/3 cup all-purpose flour
1/4 teaspoon black pepper
1 tablespoon Worcestershire sauce
1 cup low sodium chicken broth
1 cup 1% low-fat milk
3 cups of cooked white rice
2 cups diced chicken, cooked
1 cup sliced fresh mushrooms
1 tablespoon Mrs. Dash® Herb Seasoning Blend

Instructions:

1. Heat the oven to 350 degrees Fahrenheit. Spray oil-free half-quart baking dish with nonstick cooking spray.
2. Chop the bell pepper and onion.
3. In a large saucepan, heat the olive oil and butter over low heat.
4. After the butter melts, add the flour and black pepper. Cook over low heat, stirring until mixture is clean and bubbly. Remove from the heat.
5. Add Worcestershire sauce, broth, and milk. Heat until boiling, stirring continuously. Boil and stir for a minute.
6. Add cooked rice, chicken, mushrooms, bell pepper, onion, and Mrs. Dash Herb Seasoning.
7. Pour into a baking dish. Cover and bake for 30 minutes. Remove the hood and cook for 20 minutes.

Nutritional value:
- Energy value: 190Kcal
- Proteins: 5 g
- Carbohydrates: 16 g
- Fiber: 4 g
- Sugar: 4 g
- Sodium: 5 g
- Fat: 14g
  Of which:
    - Saturated: 5 g
    - Monounsaturated: 7 g
    - Polyunsaturated: 4 g

Cholesterol: 112 mg

60. CHICKEN IN WINE SAUCE

Servings: 4

Ingredients:

8 chicken thighs, bone-in, with bones and skin
2 tablespoons canola oil
1/4 teaspoonful of fresh ground pepper
Half a cup of all-purpose white flour
4 garlic cloves, peeled and cut in half
1/2 cup of white wine
1 teaspoon Mrs. Dash® Herb Seasoning Blend, any taste

Instructions:

1. Heat the oil in a large skillet over medium heat on the stove.
2. Measure the flour and put it on a plate. If you like, you can load any of the seasoning mixes to the flour, or just the black pepper.
3. Place the chicken inside the flour and place in the hot oil. Cook until lightly browned.
4. In the same skillet, add garlic and white wine.
5. Cover and cook dinner over low heat for about 20 minutes, making sure that when a knife is inserted, the juice comes out clean, not crimson. Check the chicken periodically and pour extra wine if the pan is dry.
6. Serve the chicken topped with wine sauce

Nutritional value:
- Energy value: 250 Kcal
- Proteins: 7g
- Carbohydrates: 12 g
- Fiber: 4 g
- Sugar: 4 g
- Sodium: 5 g
- Fat: 12 g
  Of which:
    - Saturated: 5 g
    - Monounsaturated: 7 g
    - Polyunsaturated: 4 g

Cholesterol: 110 mg

61. EASY LEMON CRISPY CHICKEN

Servings: 4

Ingredients:

4 cups of cooked white rice
1 pound boneless, skinless breasts
1 teaspoon herb seasoning mix
1/4 teaspoon of salt
1/4 teaspoon black pepper
1 large egg
2 teaspoons of water
1/2 cup of all-purpose white flour
2 tablespoons olive oil
4 medium lemons
2 tablespoons of chopped parsley to decorate

Instructions:

1. Prepare rice according to package directions, omitting salt.
2. Cut a lemon into 6 wedges to use as a garnish. Cut the 4 lemons in half.
3. Cut the chicken into finger-shaped slices
4. Season with herb seasonings, salt, and pepper.
5. In a medium bowl, beat the egg and water until just combined.
6. Dip the bird in eggs and then in flour. Make sure to coat both sides with flour.
7. Heat the olive oil in a nonstick skillet.
8. Sauté chicken in the skillet until golden brown on both sides. If you prefer, sauté with lemon wedges for flavor and garnish. Be careful now not to over-cook the poultry.
9. Squeeze the 6 lemon halves over the bird during sautéing.

10. Just before removing the chicken from the pan, squeeze the remaining drops of lemon juice over the bird.
11. Take the bird out of the pan. Blot excess oil from the bird with paper towels to keep it crisp.
12. Divide the birds into 4 servings and place each serving on top of 2/3 cups of white rice.
13. Garnish the chicken and rice with lemon wedges and fresh parsley.

> **Nutritional value:**
> - Energy value: 192 Kcal
> - Proteins: 19 g
> - Carbohydrates: 15 g
> - Fiber: 7 g
> - Sugar: 3 g
> - Sodium: 3 g
> - Fats: 10 g
>   - *Of which:*
>   - Saturated: 5 g
>   - Monounsaturated: 3 g
>   - Polyunsaturated: 1 g
> - Cholesterol: 127 mg

62. EASY TURKEY SLOPPY JOES

Servings: 4
Ingredients:

1/2 cup of crimson onion
1/2 cup of inexperienced bell pepper
2 kilos of ground turkey, 7% fat
1 tablespoon roast chicken mix seasoning
2 tablespoons brown sugar
1 tablespoon Worcestershire sauce
1 cup low sodium tomato sauce
6 hamburger buns

Instructions:
1. Chop the onion and bell pepper.
2. Place in a large skillet with the turkey and cook over medium-high heat until the turkey is cooked through. Do not drain.
3. In a small bowl, combine the seasoning, sugar, Worcestershire sauce, and tomato sauce.
4. Add seasonings to the turkey additive. Reduce heat to simmer and cook dinner for 10 minutes.
5. Divide into 6 batches and serve on hamburger buns.

> **Nutritional value:**
> - Energy value: 227 Kcal
> - Proteins: 5 g
> - Carbohydrates: 7 g
> - Fiber: 5 g
> - Sugar: 3 g
> - Sodium: 2 g
> - Fat: 9 g
>   - *Of which:*
>   - Saturated: 7 g
>   - Monounsaturated: 1 g
>   - Polyunsaturated: 1 g
> - Cholesterol: 100 mg

63. CLAY POT CHICKEN

Servings: 4
Ingredients:

4 kilos of complete bird
2 teaspoons Mrs. Dash Herb Seasoning Mix
1 teaspoon black pepper
1 teaspoon garlic powder

Instructions:
1. Wash the chicken and remove the giblets inside.
2. In a small bowl, combine the seasoning mix, pepper, and garlic powder.
3. Sprinkle half of the seasonings on the chicken. Rub the remaining seasoning on the outside of the bird.
4. Place the chicken bun face up in an oval crock pot or neck up in a round crock pot.
5. Cover and cook dinner over low heat for 8 hours.
6. Remove the constriction from the bones and discard the skin.

> **Nutritional value:**
> - Energy value: 260 Kcal
> - Proteins: 5 g
> - Carbohydrates: 16 g
> - Fiber: 4 g
> - Sugar: 4 g
> - Sodium: 5 g
> - Fat: 18 g
>   - *Of which:*
>   - Saturated: 5 g
>   - Monounsaturated: 7 g
>   - Polyunsaturated: 4 g
> - Cholesterol: 119 mg

64. GRILLED BUTTERMILK GARLIC MARINATED CHICKEN

Servings: 4
Ingredients:

1 cup of buttermilk
1 tablespoon of olive oil
6 cloves of garlic
1 teaspoon black pepper
2 poultry breasts, bone-in, with pores and skin (or 4 chicken thighs)

Instructions:
1. Chop the garlic cloves.
2. To make the marinade, add buttermilk, olive oil, garlic, and black pepper to a huge zippered bag. Seal bag and shake to combine the ingredients.
3. Place chicken in buttermilk marinade, seal bag and shake to distribute evenly.
4. Refrigerate the bird for at least 2 hours or up to 24 hours.
5. Preheat a grill to medium heat. Remove the chicken from the marinade and grill area. Discard the extra marinade. Grill the chicken until the internal temperature reaches 165 degrees Fahrenheit.

> **Nutritional value:**
> - Energy value: 153 Kcal
> - Proteins: 7 g
> - Carbohydrates: 16 g
> - Fiber: 7 g
> - Sugar: 5 g
> - Sodium: 2 g
> - Fats: 13 g
>   - *Of which:*
>   - Saturated: 4 g
>   - Monounsaturated: 6 g
>   - Polyunsaturated: 2 g
>
> Cholesterol: 115 mg

DESSERTS

65. CHOCOLATE PEANUT BUTTER MUFFINS

Servings: 4
Ingredients:

1/2 cup of butter
1/2 cup of honey
1/2 cup of unsweetened cocoa powder
3/4 cup creamy peanut butter
4 massive eggs
1/2 teaspoon of baking soda
3/4 cup chocolate chips

Instructions:

1. Preheat the oven to 350 degrees Fahrenheit. Line a muffin tin with parchment paper.
2. Melt the butter and honey together. Beat the cocoa powder and peanut butter until smooth.
3. Beat in the eggs and baking soda. Stir in the chocolate chips. Pour some into the muffin pan.
4. Bake for 18–22 minutes or until a toothpick inserted in the middle comes out clean.

Nutritional value:
- Energy value: 123 Kcal
- Proteins: 5 g
- Carbohydrates: 11 g
- Fiber: 4 g
- Sugar: 3 g
- Sodium: 3 g
- Fats: 13 g
  - **Of which:**
    - Saturated: 4 g
    - Monounsaturated: 6 g
    - Polyunsaturated: 2 g
- Cholesterol: 115 mg

66. BRIE AND BLUEBERRY CHUTNEY

Servings: 4
Ingredients:

12 ounces blueberries, fresh
1/2 cup sugar
1/2 cup brown sugar
1/3 cup water
1 teaspoon mustard powder
1 teaspoon garlic cloves
A pinch of cinnamon
1 teaspoon nutmeg
1 teaspoon ground allspice
8 ounces Brie cheese
30 low sodium crackers

Instructions:

1. Preheat the oven to 350 degrees Fahrenheit. Fresh blueberries should be washed and drained.
2. Heat the water in a skillet over medium heat for 5 minutes before adding the fresh blueberries. Heat for just 5 minutes, or before the blueberries start to pop.
3. Combine the white and brown sugars (or Splenda).
4. Add the spices gently.
5. Remove the pan from the heat. Let the hot sauce cool.
6. Remove Brie cheese from its packaging. Cut a circle across the top of the wheel, leaving a half-inch rim of crust, and lift the crust up from the middle to reveal the Brie inside.
7. Place brie cheese on a baking sheet and bake until cheese is soft to the touch and slightly melted on top.
8. Remove the brie cheese from the oven and place it on a serving platter.
9. Serve brie cheese with warm chutney and a selection of low sodium crackers.

Nutritional value:
- Energy value: 160 Kcal
- Proteins: 5 g
- Carbohydrates: 14 g
- Fiber: 4 g
- Sugar: 4 g
- Sodium: 3 g
- Fat: 14 g
  - **Of which:**
    - Saturated: 5 g
    - Monounsaturated: 7 g
    - Polyunsaturated: 4 g
- Cholesterol: 109 mg

67. FIG AND GOAT CHEESE CROSTINI

Servings: 2
Ingredients:

1 baguette
1 tablespoon unsalted butter
1/4 cup of extra virgin olive oil
1/2 cup crumbled goat cheese
1/2 cup canned figs or spread
Glaze made with 2 tablespoons balsamic vinegar

Instructions:

1. Preheat the oven to 375 degrees Fahrenheit. Cut the baguette into 24 1/2-inch thick slices.
2. Melt the butter and add the olive oil to make the crostini. Place each slice of bread on a baking sheet and spread the butter mixture on both sides.
3. Preheat the oven to 350 degrees Fahrenheit and bake the crostini for 5–7 minutes. Flip the slices and bake for another 5 minutes, or until golden brown and crisp.
4. On each crostini, sprinkle 1 teaspoon of figs for spread. Sprinkle 1 teaspoon of crumbled goat cheese on top. Drizzle the balsamic vinegar glaze over the crostini until they are all together.

Nutritional value:
- Energy value: 192 Kcal
- Proteins: 19 g
- Carbohydrates: 15 g
- Fiber: 7 g
- Sugar: 3 g
- Sodium: 3 g
- Fats: 10 g
  - **Of which:**
    - Saturated: 5 g
    - Monounsaturated: 3 g
    - Polyunsaturated: 1 g
- Cholesterol: 127 mg

68. APPLE MUFFINS

Servings: 2
Ingredients:

1 pound of sugar
2 large eggs

1/3 cup canola oil
1/2 teaspoon ground cinnamon
1/2 teaspoon ground ginger
1/2 teaspoon ground cloves
1/2 teaspoon nutmeg
1/4 teaspoon salt
1 teaspoon of baking soda
1 cup unsweetened applesauce
2 cups all-purpose flour
1 medium apple

Instructions:

1. Preheat the oven to 325 degrees Fahrenheit.
2. With nonstick cooking spray, grease a muffin pan.
3. Combine the sugar, oil, and eggs in a mixing bowl.
4. Mix together the spices, salt, baking soda, and applesauce.
5. Add the flour until a thick dough forms.
6. Cut the apple into small pieces by slicing or chopping (peel if desired).
7. Place a small tablespoon of batter in the bottom of each muffin tin, place slices, and top with more batter if using slices. If you are using apple chunks, mix them into the batter before filling the muffin cups.
8. Preheat oven to 350 degrees Fahrenheit and bake for 25–30 minutes, or until firm to the touch. Remove from oven and let cool.

Nutritional value:
- Energy value: 180 Kcal
- Proteins: 5 g
- Carbohydrates: 15 g
- Fiber: 4 g
- Sugar: 4 g
- Sodium: 3 g
- Fat: 13 g
  Of which:
  - Saturated: 5 g
  - Monounsaturated: 7 g
  - Polyunsaturated: 4 g

Cholesterol: 114 mg

69. ANGELINA'S GINGERBREAD MUFFINS

Servings: 2
Ingredients:
2 large eggs
3/4 cup low-fat milk (1% fat)
6 tablespoons canola oil
1/2 cup of brown sugar, well packed
4 tablespoons corn syrup (dark)
2 cups all-purpose flour
1 teaspoon baking soda powder
4 teaspoons ground ginger
1 1/2 teaspoons ground cinnamon

Instructions:

1. Preheat the oven to 400 degrees Fahrenheit. Grease or line a 12-cup muffin tin with paper liners.
2. Lightly beat the eggs in a medium bowl. Combine milk, oil, brown sugar, and corn syrup in a bowl.
3. Combine flour, baking powder, ginger, and cinnamon in a large mixing bowl. Pour the liquid ingredients into a well in the middle of the dry ingredients. Don't over mix. Stir gently until blended.
4. Fill muffin pan half full with batter. Bake for about 20 minutes, or until golden brown and firm to the touch in a preheated oven.

5. Remove the muffins from the oven and cool for 5 minutes in the pan. Serve with a tablespoon of butter or cream cheese on top.

Nutritional value:
- Energy value: 153 Kcal
- Proteins: 7 g
- Carbohydrates: 16 g
- Fiber: 7 g
- Sugar: 5 g
- Sodium: 2 g
- Fats: 13 g
  Of which:
  - Saturated: 4 g
  - Monounsaturated: 6 g
  - Polyunsaturated: 2 g
- Cholesterol: 115 mg

70. APPLE PIE

Servings: 4
Ingredients:
6 apples, medium
1/2 cup sugar (granulated)
1 teaspoon ground cinnamon
6 tablespoons butter
2 1/3 cup all-purpose flour
1 pound of vegetable shortening
6 tablespoons water

Instructions:

1. Preheat the oven to 425 degrees Fahrenheit.
2. Apples should be peeled, cored, and sliced.
3. Combine apple slices, sugar, and cinnamon in a large mixing bowl. Set aside, covered.
4. Using a pastry mixer, cut the shortening into flour in a separate large bowl. 1 tablespoon at a time, add cold water and mix until dough forms a ball. If not, roll your hands into a ball.
5. Divide the dough in half and roll out the half with a rolling pin and more flour if necessary. Fill 9" pie pan halfway with batter.
6. Fill the peel halfway with the apple pie filling.
7. Spoon 1 tablespoon of butter around the edge of pie filling, evenly distributed.
8. Roll out the remaining half of the dough. Place on top of the apple pie filling, making sure the edges of the pie are covered.
9. Make four 1" cuts around the bottom of the cake with a sharp knife to allow air to escape while baking.
10. Place the tart in a jelly pan in the oven to collect the juices while it bakes.
11. Preheat the oven to 350 degrees Fahrenheit and bake for 50 to 60 minutes, or until the base is golden brown.

Nutritional value:
- Energy value: 190 Kcal
- Proteins: 5 g
- Carbohydrates: 15 g
- Fiber: 4 g
- Sugar: 4 g
- Sodium: 3 g
- Fat: 18 g
  Of which:
  - Saturated: 5 g
  - Monounsaturated: 7 g
  - Polyunsaturated: 4 g

Cholesterol: 117 mg

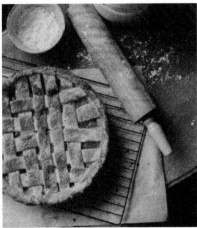

71. FROZEN GRAPES

Servings: 4
Ingredients:
5 cups of grapes (without seeds)
3 ounces flavored gelatin
Instructions:
1. The grapes should be washed and destemmed but left slightly damp.
2. In a large bowl, pour the dry gelatin mixture. Do not use water to dissolve.
3. Toss the wet grapes in the bowl to coat them evenly.
4. Arrange the coated grapes on a baking sheet in a single layer or flatten them in a plastic bag with a sealed lid.
5. The grapes must be frozen for at least an hour. Relax and enjoy.

Nutritional value:
- Energy value: 260 Kcal
- Proteins: 5 g
- Carbohydrates: 16 g
- Fiber: 4 g
- Sugar: 4 g
- Sodium: 5 g
- Fat: 18 g
  Of which:
  - Saturated: 5 g
  - Monounsaturated: 7 g
  - Polyunsaturated: 4 g
- Cholesterol: 119 mg

72. CRAN-APPLE AND CINNAMON SNACK MIX

Servings: 3
Ingredients:
1 cup apples (dried)
2 cups of corn chicken food
2 cups Chex® Shredded Wheat Spoon Size Cereal
3 cups of Cinnamon Chex® Cereal
1 cup dried cranberries, sweetened
1/4 cup of liquid egg whites
2 tablespoons apple juice
1/2 cup sugar
A pinch of cinnamon
1 tablespoon sesame beans
Instructions:
1. Preheat the oven to 300 degrees Fahrenheit. Nonstick cooking spray for large rectangular cake pan (9x13" or larger).
2. Dice the dried apples.
3. Combine cereal and dried fruit in a large mixing bowl; set aside.
4. Using a mixer or hand mixer, beat the egg whites, sugar, apple juice, and cinnamon until frothy in a medium bowl.
5. Stir the egg mixture into the cereal in the bowl until evenly coated.
6. Sesame seeds can be sprinkled on top.
7. Bake for 45 minutes, stirring every 15 minutes, or until cereal is lightly browned and crisp.
8. Let cool absolutely. Keep the jar airtight.

Nutritional value:
- Energy value: 175 Kcal
- Proteins: 13 g
- Carbohydrates: 11 g
- Fiber: 3 g
- Sugar: 2 g
- Sodium: 3 g
- Fats: 11 g
  Of which:
  - Saturated: 3 g
  - Monounsaturated: 5 g
  - Polyunsaturated: 2 g

Cholesterol: 87 mg

BASES

73. FLOUR TORTILLAS

Servings: 3

Ingredients:

6 cups all-purpose white flour
1 teaspoon salt
1 cup shortening, softened
2-1/4 cups warm water

Instructions:

1. In a large bowl, mix together the flour and salt.
2. Add soft butter and 2 cups of warm water.
3. Begin mixing by hand, squeezing out the flour and shortening with your fingers or mixing with a spoon and knife, crisscrossing the flour and shortening.
4. Shape the dough into a large ball. Remove adhering flour from the sides of the bowl by rolling the dough around the bowl. Add remaining 1/4 cup warm water if the batter is too dry.
5. Place the dough on a board or table and knead for a minute until you get a smooth ball. Cover with the bowl or towel for at least 5 minutes and let it rest.
6. Start heating a cast iron griddle or heavy skillet to medium-high heat.
7. Pinch a piece of dough into a 2-inch round ball, flipping the edges of the dough down and inward. Put each ball aside. They will feel dry to the touch.
8. Sprinkle flour lightly over the dough and the board or tabletop. Using a rolling pin, roll the dough into a round tortilla about 6 to 7 inches in diameter.
9. Mix and flip the tortilla between your hands until smooth.
10. Try a small piece of dough on a hot griddle or skillet; It should start to brown in a few seconds if the oil is hot enough.
11. Cook each tortilla until lightly browned on both sides, turning frequently to avoid burning. Use a spatula or tongs to turn the tortillas.
12. Stack the tortillas after cooking. Let cool before storing.

Nutritional value:
- Energy value: 192 Kcal
- Proteins: 19 g
- Carbohydrates: 15 g
- Fiber: 7 g
- Sugar: 3 g
- Sodium: 3 g
- Fats: 10 g
  Of which:
  - Saturated: 5 g
  - Monounsaturated: 3 g
  - Polyunsaturated: 1 g

Cholesterol: 127 mg

74. EASY SEASONING DIP WITHOUT SALT

Servings: 1

Ingredients:

1/2 cup Greek yogurt (fat-free)
1/2 cup of sour cream
1 1/2 teaspoons herb seasoning mix (unsalted)
1 teaspoon reduced-sodium Worcestershire sauce

Instructions:

1. Combine all ingredients in a small mixing bowl.

2. To allow the flavor to develop, cover and chill for at least 4 hours.
3. Until serving, stir well.

Nutritional value:
- Energy value: 227 Kcal
- Proteins: 5 g
- Carbohydrates: 7 g
- Fiber: 5 g
- Sugar: 3 g
- Sodium: 2 g
- Fat: 9 g
  Of which:
  - Saturated: 7 g
  - Monounsaturated: 1 g
  - Polyunsaturated: 1 g
- Cholesterol: 100 mg

75. APPLE ZUCCHINI BREAD

Servings: 4

Ingredients:

3/4 cups plus 2 tablespoons all-purpose flour
1 cup Granny Smith apples
2 cups of zucchini
4 large eggs
1/2 cup of vegetable oil
3/4 cup granulated sugar
1 cup of brown sugar
1 teaspoon vanilla extract
1 1/2 teaspoons of baking soda
1/2 teaspoon of salt
3 teaspoons ground cinnamon
2 tablespoons unsalted butter

Instructions:

1. Preheat oven to 350 degrees Fahrenheit. Grease and flour two 9x 5" loaf pans with 2 tablespoons flour.
2. Peel and chop the apples; grate the zucchini.
3. In a large bowl, combine the eggs, oil, granulated sugar, 3/4 cup brown sugar (or 6 tablespoons Splenda® Brown Sugar Mix), and vanilla.
4. In a separate large bowl, mix baking soda, 3 1/2 cups of flour, salt, and a couple of teaspoons of cinnamon.
5. Add the flour to the egg mixture. Now, don't over mix.
6. Add the apples and zucchini and pour the mixture into loaf pans. Spread the combination lightly.
7. Bake for 40 minutes.
8. While the bread is baking, make the crumb topping: combine the last 1/4 cup flour, 1/4 cup brown sugar (or 2 tablespoons Splenda® brown sugar mixture), and 1 teaspoon cinnamon. Cut the butter until the aggregate becomes very crumbly.
9. Remove the bread from the oven as soon as it has baked for 40 minutes and add the crumb topping.
10. Bake for 10 more minutes or until the toothpick comes out soft (from the center of the loaf).
11. Let cool for 10 minutes, then remove loaves from pans and transfer to wire racks to cool completely.
12. Cut all loaves into 18-1/2 slices before serving.

Nutritional value:
- Energy value: 260 Kcal
- Proteins: 5 g
- Carbohydrates: 16 g
- Fiber: 4 g
- Sugar: 4 g
- Sodium: 5 g

- Fat: 18 g
  - *Of which:*
    - o   Saturated: 5 g
    - o   Monounsaturated: 7 g
    - o   Polyunsaturated: 4 g
- Cholesterol: 119 mg

76. CRANBERRY NUT BREAD

Servings: 4
Ingredients:

1 half cups cleaned cranberries
2 cups all-purpose flour
1 cup of sugar
1/2 teaspoons baking powder
1/2 teaspoon of baking soda
1 large egg
1/2 cup of cranberry juice or apple juice
1 teaspoon orange zest
2 tablespoons margarine
1/4 cup walnuts, chopped
2 tablespoons of hot water

Instructions:

1. Cut each blueberry in half and reserve.
2. Preheat the oven to 350 degrees Fahrenheit. Grease a loaf pan and cover with wax paper. Grease the waxed paper. Set aside.
3. Sift the flour, sugar, baking powder, and baking soda into a large bowl.
4. In a separate bowl, combine the juice, orange zest, melted margarine, and crushed egg. Add to the flour mix and simply stir until flour is mixed.
5. Mix with the blueberries and walnuts. Add hot water.
6. Place the dough in a prepared loaf pan and bake for 1 hour 10 minutes. Try inserting a toothpick into the bread; if it comes out easy the bread is made.
7. Chill the bread in the pan for 10 minutes, then leave it and put it on a rack. Cut into 10 slices.

Nutritional value:
- Energy value: 192 Kcal
- Proteins: 19 g
- Carbohydrates: 15 g
- Fiber: 7 g
- Sugar: 3 g
- Sodium: 3 g
- Fats: 10 g
  - *Of which:*
    - o   Saturated: 5 g
    - o   Monounsaturated: 3 g
    - o   Polyunsaturated: 1 g
- Cholesterol: 127 mg

77. CLOUD BREAD

Servings: 3
Ingredients:

6 large eggs
1/2 teaspoon cream of tartar
3/4 cup sour cream
1/2 teaspoon of baking powder
1/8 teaspoon salt
1/2 cup of whey protein powder

Instructions:

1. Preheat the oven to 300 degrees Fahrenheit. Separate the eggs, setting the yolks aside for later.
2. Using a stand or hand mixer, beat the egg whites and cream of tartar until stiff peaks form. Set aside.
3. Mix the egg yolks in a bowl with the Ingredients: Finishes and stir well to combine.

4. Using a small number of egg whites, gently fold in the yolk addition one touch at a time until well combined. Continue adding final egg whites.
5. Pour the mixture into a greased loaf pan.
6. Bake in the center of the oven for fifty to 60 minutes, until a toothpick inserted into the center, comes out easily.
7. Let the cloud bread cool. Remove from the pan and slice. Store in the refrigerator.

Nutritional value:
- Energy value: 153 Kcal
- Proteins: 7 g
- Carbohydrates: 16 g
- Fiber: 7 g
- Sugar: 5 g
- Sodium: 2 g
- Fats: 13 g
  - *Of which:*
    - o   Saturated: 4 g
    - o   Monounsaturated: 6 g
    - o   Polyunsaturated: 2 g
- Cholesterol: 115 mg

78. COCONUT BREAD

Servings: 2
Ingredients:

2 tablespoons coconut oil
1/3 cup unsalted butter
1/2 cup of sugar
2 large eggs
1 cup of grated coconut, dried and sweetened
1 cup sour cream
2 cups of all-purpose flour
1 teaspoon of baking soda
1/2 teaspoons baking powder

Instructions:

1. Preheat the oven to 350 degrees Fahrenheit. Grease a 9x5-inch loaf pan. Put the butter so that it melts.
2. Heat the coconut oil in the microwave until it evaporates. Set aside to cool.
3. Beat in the butter and sugar. Add the coconut oil and eggs; stir collectively. Stir in the sour cream. Add grated coconut to the mixture and stir.
4. In a separate bowl, mix together the flour, baking soda, and baking powder.
5. Fold the dry ingredients into the wet ingredients. Pour the batter into the loaf pan.
6. Bake for 45 to 60 minutes, until the bread is golden brown and a toothpick comes out clean.
7. Chill the bread in the pan for 5 to 10 minutes, then remove it from the pan and let it cool on a wire rack.

Nutritional value:
- Energy value: 160 Kcal
- Proteins: 5 g
- Carbohydrates: 18g
- Fiber: 4 g
- Sugar: 4 g
- Sodium: 5 g
- Fat: 14g
  - *Of which:*
    - o   Saturated: 5 g
    - o   Monounsaturated: 7 g
    - o   Polyunsaturated: 4 g
- Cholesterol: 119 mg

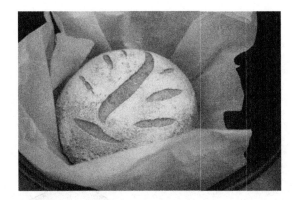

79. ARTICHOKE DIP

Servings: 1
Ingredients:

1 cup artichoke hearts, frozen
1 tablespoon of mayonnaise
1/4 cup of sour cream
2 teaspoons of cream cheese
1 large garlic clove
2 teaspoons chili sauce
1 tablespoon Parmigiano Reggiano

Instructions:

1   Preheat the oven to 375 degrees Fahrenheit.
2   In a saucepan, cover the artichoke hearts with water and bring to a boil. Reduce heat to medium and continue cooking for another 6 minutes. Cool, drain, and rinse with cold water.
3   Chop the artichoke hearts into small pieces.
4   Combine the mayonnaise, sour cream, cream cheese, hot sauce, and crushed garlic clove in a medium cup. Add the artichoke hearts until well combined. Fill a baking dish halfway with the mixture.
5   Parmesan cheese should be sprinkled on top. Preheat in the oven to 350 degrees Fahrenheit and bake for 30 minutes, or until the top is bubbly.

Nutritional value:
• Energy value: 192 Kcal
• Proteins: 19 g
• Carbohydrates: 15 g
• Fiber: 7 g
• Sugar: 3 g
• Sodium: 3 g
• Fats: 10 g
Of which:
o   Saturated: 5 g
o   Monounsaturated: 3 g
o   Polyunsaturated: 1 g
• Cholesterol: 127 mg

80.   BEAN DIP

Servings: 4
Ingredients:

1 red onion, minced
1 green bell pepper
1 red bell pepper, chopped
1/3 cup cilantro, chopped
2-1/2 cups cooked white ground corn (canned or fresh)
1 cup cooked fresh pinto beans
12 ounces cream cheese (low fat)
1/4 cup of extra-virgin olive oil
3 garlic cloves
1 tablespoon ground cumin
1/4 teaspoon chili powder
12 ounces sour cream (low fat)

Instructions:

1   Chop the onion, bell peppers, and cilantro into small pieces.

2   In a food processor, combine the ground corn, pinto beans, low-fat cream cheese, olive oil, 2 garlic cloves, cumin, and optional chili powder. Pour into a 9x9" baking pan.
3   Spread a layer of sour cream over the bean mixture with a spatula.
4   In a skillet, lightly sauté the red onion, green and red bell peppers, and 1 clove of garlic. To keep peppers strong and not mushy, don't overcook them.
5   For added flavor, squeeze lime over the sautéed bell pepper and onion mixture, then squeeze out excess liquid.
6   Smooth pepper mixture over sour cream until completely covered.

Nutritional value:
• Energy value: 190 Kcal
• Proteins: 5 g
• Carbohydrates: 15 g
• Fiber: 4 g
• Sugar: 4 g
• Sodium: 3 g
• Fat: 15 g
Of which:
o   Saturated: 5 g
o   Monounsaturated: 7 g
o   Polyunsaturated: 4 g
Cholesterol: 115mg

81. BUFFALO CHICKEN DIP

Servings: 2
Ingredients:

4 ounces cream cheese
1/2 cup roasted red bell peppers, bottled
1 cup sour cream (low-fat)
4 teaspoons Tabasco® hot pepper sauce
2 cups cooked chicken, shredded

Instructions:

1   Let the cream cheese melt in the refrigerator.
2   Measure out 1/2 cup of red bell peppers after drying. To produce red pepper sauce, puree in a blender or food processor.
3   Beat cream cheese and sour cream in a medium bowl until smooth. 2 teaspoons of Tabasco sauce plus pepper puree. Stir until well mixed.
4   Gently fold the chicken. Add more hot sauce if you like. 1/2 teaspoon at a time; taste and adjust the hot sauce to the desired amount of heat.
5   Cook for 2 to 3 hours over low heat in a slow cooker, or bake for 30 minutes at 350 degrees Fahrenheit in the oven.
6   Serve warm sauce with carrots, celery, cucumber, and cauliflower for dipping, or top the sauce with lettuce leaves or cabbage to make mini rolls.

Nutritional value:
• Energy value: 175 Kcal
• Proteins: 13 g
• Carbohydrates: 11 g
• Fiber: 3 g
• Sugar: 2 g
• Sodium: 3 g
• Fats: 11 g
Of which:
o   Saturated: 3 g
o   Monounsaturated: 5 g
o   Polyunsaturated: 2 g
• Cholesterol: 87 mg

82. APPLE CINNAMON BREAD

Servings: 2
Ingredients:

1/2 cup unsalted butter
1 large apple
1/2 cup medium packed brown sugar

1-1/2 teaspoon ground cinnamon
2/3 cup granulated sugar
2 large eggs
2 teaspoons vanilla extract
1-1/2 cups all-purpose flour
1-1/2 tablespoons baking powder
1/2 cup of milk

Instructions:

1. Preheat the oven to 350 degrees Fahrenheit. Place the butter to soften. Grease a 9x5-inch loaf pan. Peel and finely chop the apple.
2. In a mug, combine brown sugar and cinnamon; set aside.
3. Combine granulated sugar and butter in a stand mixer and beat until smooth.
4. Continue beating on medium speed until the eggs and vanilla are completely combined.
5. Add the flour and baking powder until well combined. Add the milk to the dough.
6. Half of the dough should be poured into the loaf pan, followed by half of the chopped apples and half of the cinnamon and sugar mixture. Pour the remaining batter on top. With the back of a spoon, gently press down on the apples remaining in the dough. Apply the rest of the cinnamon and sugar mixture on top once more.
7. Bake for 45 to 55 minutes, or until a toothpick inserted in the middle comes out clean. Cool in the loaf pan for 10 minutes before transferring to a wire rack to cool.
8. Cut the bread into twelve 3/4-inch slices once it has cooled.

Nutritional value:
- Energy value: 260 Kcal
- Proteins: 6 g
- Carbohydrates: 18 g
- Fiber: 4 g
- Sugar: 4 g
- Sodium: 4 g
- Fat: 16 g
  Of which:
  - Saturated: 5 g
  - Monounsaturated: 7 g
  - Polyunsaturated: 4 g

Cholesterol: 118 mg

83. ARTICHOKE DRESSING ON TOASTED PITA

Servings: 4
Ingredients:

14 ounces artichoke hearts, canned
2 ounces diced bell pepper in a can
2 onions (green)
1 garlic clove
3 tablespoons grated Parmesan cheese
2 tablespoons lemon juice
1 tablespoon of extra virgin olive oil
1/2 teaspoon of pepper
4 rounds of 7-inch pita bread

Instructions:

1. The artichoke hearts and bell pepper should be drained and minced. Green onions should be thinly sliced, and the garlic clove should be minced.
2. In a bowl, combine all ingredients except the pitas and stir well.
3. Chill 8 hours or overnight, covered.
4. Preheat the oven to 350 degrees Fahrenheit.
5. Open the pita slices by cutting them in half. Make 8 wedges by cutting each half into chunks.
6. Place the pita slices, smooth side down, on a baking sheet and spray with cooking spray. Preheat oven to 350 degrees Fahrenheit and bake for 8 minutes, or until lightly browned.
7. Let the pita slices cool completely before storing them in an airtight container until ready to use.
8. Pour 1 tablespoon artichoke sauce on top of each pita wedge.

Nutritional value:
- Energy value: 160 Kcal
- Proteins: 5 g
- Carbohydrates: 17 g
- Fiber: 4 g
- Sugar: 4 g
- Sodium: 4 g
- Fat: 16 g
  Of which:
  - Saturated: 5 g
  - Monounsaturated: 7 g
  - Polyunsaturated: 4 g

Cholesterol: 119 mg

DRINKS

84. BEET AND APPLE JUICE MIX

Servings: 2

Ingredients:

1 apple (medium)
1/2 medium beet
1 medium carrot (fresh)
1 stalk of celery
1/4 cup of parsley

Instructions:

1. In a juicer, process the apple, beet, carrot, celery, and parsley to extract the juice.
2. To make two servings, pour the mixture into two small glasses. Drink immediately or chill in the refrigerator.

> **Nutritional value:**
> - Energy value: 87 Kcal
> - Proteins: 5 g
> - Carbohydrates: 11 g
> - Fiber: 3 g
> - Sugar: 2 g
> - Sodium: 2 g
> - Fats: 15 g
>   **Of which:**
>   - Saturated: 5 g
>   - Monounsaturated: 6 g
>   - Polyunsaturated: 3 g
> - Cholesterol: 157 mg

85. CARAMEL PROTEIN LATTE

Servings: 2

Ingredients:

1 apple (medium)
1/2 medium beet
1 medium carrot (fresh)
1 celery
1 heaping scoop (20.5 g) whey protein powder
2 ounces of water
2 ounces protein powder
6 ounces of freshly brewed coffee
1/4 cup DaVinci Gourmet® Sugar-Free Syrup, Caramel

Instructions:

1. In a cup, put 1 tablespoon of protein powder and then 1 tablespoon of water
2. Add 6 ounces of hot coffee.
3. Add caramel syrup with a sugar-free sweetener of your choice; adjust sweetness to taste. Prepare 1/4 cup of parsley.
4. In a juicer, process the apple, beet, carrot, celery, and parsley to extract the juice.
5. To make two servings, pour the mixture into two small glasses. Drink immediately or chill in the refrigerator.

> **Nutritional value:**
> - Energy value: 153 Kcal
> - Proteins: 7 g
> - Carbohydrates: 16 g
> - Fiber: 7 g
> - Sugar: 5 g
> - Sodium: 2 g
> - Fats: 13 g
>   **Of which:**
>   - Saturated: 4 g
>   - Monounsaturated: 6 g
>   - Polyunsaturated: 2 g
> - Cholesterol: 115 mg

86. CHOCOLATE MILKSHAKE

Servings: 2

Ingredients:

1 tablespoon unsweetened bakery cocoa powder
1 tablespoon of ice water
1 teaspoon sugar (or sugar substitute)
3 egg white (pasteurized)
4 tablespoons whipped topping
Shavings from a chocolate bar (optional)

Instructions:

1. Combine cocoa, cold water, and sugar in a bowl.
2. Stir until the sugar is completely dissolved.
3. Add 3 tablespoons whipped topping, plus 3 egg whites. Blend until all whipped topping has melted.
4. Pour 1 tablespoon whipped topping and chocolate shavings on top.

> **Nutritional value:**
> - Energy value: 260 Kcal
> - Proteins: 5 g
> - Carbohydrates: 16 g
> - Fiber: 4 g
> - Sugar: 4 g
> - Sodium: 5 g
> - Fat: 18 g
>   **Of which:**
>   - Saturated: 5 g
>   - Monounsaturated: 7 g
>   - Polyunsaturated: 4 g
> - Cholesterol: 119 mg

87. CITRUS SMOOTHIE

Servings: 1

Ingredients:

1/2 cup of pineapple juice
1/2 cup unsweetened almond milk
1 cup of orange sherbet
1/2 cup low cholesterol egg product

Instructions:

1. Blend the ingredients for 30 seconds in a blender.
2. Divide the mixture into two portions.
3. Serve immediately or save for later. Ingredients:

> **Nutritional value:**
> - Energy value: 153 Kcal
> - Proteins: 7 g
> - Carbohydrates: 16 g
> - Fiber: 7 g
> - Sugar: 5 g

- Sodium: 2 g
- Fats: 13 g
  Of which:
  - Saturated: 4 g
  - Monounsaturated: 6 g
  - Polyunsaturated: 2 g
- Cholesterol: 115 mg

88. CUCUMBER AND LEMON-FLAVORED WATER

Servings: 1
Ingredients:

1 cucumber, medium
1 lemon
1/4 cup of basil leaves
1/4 cup of fresh mint leaves
4 cups of water

Instructions:
1. Cucumber and lemon should be cut into thin slices.
2. Finely chop the basil and mint leaves.
3. In a pitcher, combine all of the ingredients.
4. Refrigerate for at least 24 hours before serving.

   Nutritional value:
   - Energy value: 227 Kcal
   - Proteins: 5 g
   - Carbohydrates: 7 g
   - Fiber: 5 g
   - Sugar: 3 g
   - Sodium: 2 g
   - Fat: 9 g
     Of which:
     - Saturated: 7 g
     - Monounsaturated: 1 g
     - Polyunsaturated: 1 g
   - Cholesterol: 100 mg

89. EASY PINEAPPLE PROTEIN SHAKE

Servings: 2
Ingredients:

3/4 cup sorbet or pineapple sorbet
1 scoop whey protein powder (vanilla)
2 ice cubes (optional)
1/2 cup water

Instructions:
1. Combine pineapple sorbet, whey protein powder, and water in a blender (ice cubes optional).
2. Blend for 30 to 45 seconds immediately.

   Nutritional value:
   - Energy value: 192 Kcal
   - Proteins: 19 g
   - Carbohydrates: 15 g
   - Fiber: 7 g
   - Sugar: 3 g
   - Sodium: 3 g
   - Fats: 10 g
     Of which:
     - Saturated: 5 g
     - Monounsaturated: 3 g
     - Polyunsaturated: 1 g
   - Cholesterol: 127 mg

90. FABULOUS HOT COCOA

Servings: 1
Ingredients:

1 cup of very hot water

1 tablespoon unsweetened cocoa powder
2 teaspoons granulated sugar
2 tablespoons cold water
3 teaspoons of whipped cream

Instructions:
1. Heat a cup of water.
2. While the water is heating, mix the cocoa powder and sugar in a cup.
3. Add cold water and mix to form a fine paste.
4. Add hot water to the mug. Stir to dissolve the paste.
5. Top with whipped cream.

   Nutritional value:
   - Energy value: 116 Kcal
   - Proteins: 5 g
   - Carbohydrates: 8 g
   - Fiber: 3 g
   - Sugar: 4 g
   - Sodium: 3 g
   - Fats: 10 g
     Of which:
     - Saturated: 3 g
     - Monounsaturated: 5 g
     - Polyunsaturated: 1 g
   - Cholesterol: 105 mg

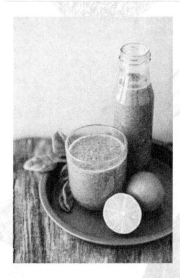

91. GREEN JUICE

Servings: 1
Ingredients:

2 apples (medium green)
1/2 lemon
1/2 cup pineapple (fresh)
1 cucumber, medium

Instructions:
1. The product must be thoroughly washed.
2. Apples must have hearts.
3. With a juicer, mix all the ingredients. Divide the mixture into two portions and enjoy!

   Nutritional value:
   - Energy value: 163 Kcal
   - Proteins: 4 g
   - Carbohydrates: 8 g
   - Fiber: 3 g
   - Sugar: 4 g
   - Sodium: 2 g
   - Fats: 11 g
     Of which:
     - Saturated: 3 g
     - Monounsaturated: 4 g

- o   Polyunsaturated: 2 g
- Cholesterol: 129 mg

92. HIGH PROTEIN RICE MILK

Servings: 1
Ingredients:

1 cup unenriched rice milk, cold
2 tablespoons whey protein (vanilla)

Instructions:
1   In a blender, combine the rice milk and protein powder and blend until smooth.
2   Divide the mixture into two portions. One to savor now and one to savor later.

> **Nutritional value:**
> - Energy value: 192 Kcal
> - Proteins: 19 g
> - Carbohydrates: 15 g
> - Fiber: 7 g
> - Sugar: 3 g
> - Sodium: 3 g
> - Fats: 10 g
>   *Of which:*
>   - o   Saturated: 5 g
>   - o   Monounsaturated: 3 g
>   - o   Polyunsaturated: 1 g
>
> Cholesterol: 127 mg

93. HIGH PROTEIN ROOT BEER FLOAT

Servings: 1
Ingredients:

1 cup of whipped topping for frozen desserts
2 scoops of whey protein powder
1/2 teaspoon vanilla extract
1 cup of root beer

Instructions:
1   Combine thawed whipped topping, protein powder, and vanilla extract in a large mixing bowl. Freeze the mixture until it is solid.
2   Place 2 tablespoons of frozen mixture into each of two 8-ounce glasses. In each glass, pour 4 ounces of chilled root beer over tablespoons of whipped topping mix.
3   Serve and have fun!

> **Nutritional value:**
> - Energy value: 127 Kcal
> - Proteins: 7 g

- Carbohydrates: 8 g
- Fiber: 3 g
- Sugar: 4 g
- Sodium: 2 g
- Fats: 12 g
  Of which:
  - o   Saturated: 5 g
  - o   Monounsaturated: 4 g
  - o   Polyunsaturated: 2 g
- Cholesterol: 113 mg

94. HOMEMADE ALMOND MILK

Servings: 3
Ingredients:

1 cup of raw almonds
3 cups filtered water plus soaking water
1 teaspoon vanilla extract

Instructions:
1   Fill a jar halfway with filtered water and add raw almonds. Soak the jar for 6 hours at room temperature or overnight in the refrigerator.
2   Place the almonds in a blender after draining them.
3   Fill the blender with 3 cups of filtered water.
4   Start blending on a low level and gradually increase to a high level. Blend for 2 minutes, or until the liquid has turned white and the almonds are finely chopped.
5   Over a bowl, place cheesecloth or a bag of walnuts. To strain the liquid from the almond flour, pour the liquid in batches. To remove the liquid, squeeze the cheesecloth or bag of nuts. Remove the almond flour and discard it.
6   If desired, add vanilla extract and other flavorings.
7   Fill a jar halfway with almond milk, cover, and keep refrigerated for up to 3 days. Before serving, shake well.

> **Nutritional value:**
> - Energy value: 89 Kcal
> - Proteins: 6 g
> - Carbohydrates: 6 g
> - Fiber: 5 g
> - Sugar: 3 g
> - Sodium: 3 g
> - Fat: 9 g
>   *Of which:*
>   - o   Saturated: 3 g
>   - o   Monounsaturated: 4 g
>   - o   Polyunsaturated: 1 g
> - Cholesterol: 61 mg

RENAL PLAN

WEEK N° 1

Monday	Breakfast:
	  – 9 oz chorizo omelet with eggs
	  – 2 slices of toast
	  – 1 glass of natural papaya juice
	  – 1 slice of unsalted cheese
	Snack:
	  – 1 yogurt with fruit: apple or blueberry
	Lunch:
	  – 9 oz Crock-Pot Oriental Chicken
	  – 1 cup carrot, purple cabbage, and onion salad
	  – ½ cup mashed potatoes
	Afternoon snack:
	  – 1 cup of fruit salad: banana, mango, and melon. (Additional you can add 1 tablespoon of oats)
	Dinner:
	  – A green juice

Tuesday	Breakfast:
	  – Make an easy dip with fruits for the summer
	  – ½ cup of apple or banana
	  – 1 glass of oatmeal
	Snack:
	  – A blueberry smoothie
	Lunch:
	  – 4 oz autumn wild rice
	  – 1 glass of melon juice
	Afternoon snack:
	  – 1 Chocolate Peanut Butter Muffins
	  – 1 cup of tea (ginger, cinnamon, or green tea)
	Dinner:
	  – 9 oz meat "Low Protein Hamburger Brewery"
	  – 1/2 cup Caesar salad
	  – A glass of melon juice

Wednesday	Breakfast:
	  – 2 apple toasts
	  – 2 small slices of unsalted cheese
	  – ½ of melon cut into pieces
	  – Fabulous Hot Cocoa
	Snack:
	  – 5 oz Apple Cinnamon Maple Granola
	Dinner:
	  – 5 oz of Cold Veggie Pizza Sandwiches
	  – 1 glass of carrot juice with beetroot

Thursday	Breakfast:
	  – 9 oz of Dilly Scrambled Eggs
	  – 2 slices of toast
	  – Cream cheese without salt
	  – 1 glass of homemade almond milk
	  – 4½ oz of cut fruits
	Snack:
	  – 1 acai berry smoothie
	Lunch:
	  – 5 oz of barbecued meatballs
	  – 5 oz of Asparagus Spread
	  – 1 glass of natural juice (except citrus)
	Afternoon snack:
	  – 1 Addictive Pretzel

	– 1 cup of tea *Dinner:* – 3–4 falafel of 1 oz each – Carrot, beet, and onion salad – 1 glass of natural juice
Friday	*Breakfast:* – Apple and onion omelet – 2 toasted slices of bread with margarine and garlic – 1 glass of natural juice *Snack:* – Caramel Protein Latte *Lunch:* – 5 oz of Bagel with Egg and Salmon – 4½ oz mashed potato – Raw salad of lettuce, cucumber, onion, and tomato *Afternoon snack:* – Chocolate peanut butter muffins – 1 cup of tea or coffee *Dinner:* – 2 flour tortillas – 5 oz of vegetables cut in julienne and sautéed (carrot, pods, zucchini, paprika) – Beet and apple juice mix
Saturday	*Breakfast:* – 2 cloud bread – Buffalo Chicken Dip – Beet and apple juice mix *Snack:* – 1 glass of easy pineapple protein shake *Lunch:* – 5 oz of chicken squares – 4 oz of rustic potatoes – 5 oz of cucumber, tomato, and onion salad *Afternoon snack:* – Angelina's Gingerbread Muffins – Cup of tea *Dinner:* – 5 oz artichoke dressing on toasted pita – 1 glass of citrus smoothie
Sunday	*Breakfast:* – 5 oz breakfast casserole – 2 toasts of bread – Easy Summer Fruit Dip Spread – 1 glass of homemade almond milk *Snack:* – 1 cup frozen grapes *Lunch:* – 5 oz crock pot chicken – Cucumber, carrot, onion, and tomato salad *Afternoon snack:* – Fig and Goat Cheese Crostini – 1 cup of tea *Dinner:* – 2 meat tacos – Tomato, onion, and coriander salad 1 glass of citrus juice

WEEK N° 2

Monday	Lunch: – 1 spice cutlet with apple – Vegetable salad – 1 cup of rice Snack: – Cran-apple and cinnamon sandwich mix Dinner: – 1 easy chicken and pasta dinner plate – 1 glass of green juice
Tuesday	Breakfast: – 2 Belgian Waffles – A glass of high protein rice milk Snack: – A glass of green juice Lunch: – ½ Roast Chicken Breast, Asparagus, and Corn – Striped carrot and beet salad, with onion and coriander – Zucchini croquettes Afternoon snack: – 1 portion or 4 oz standing apple – A cup of coffee Dinner: – 2 flour tortillas – 4½ oz of Buffalo Chicken Dip
Wednesday	Breakfast: – 4½ oz Apple Cinnamon French Toast Strata – 5 oz of buffalo chicken dip Snack: – 1 glass of green juice Lunch: – 4½ oz braised beef ribs – 5 oz stir-fry mixed vegetables – ½ cup of green rice Afternoon snack: – A serving of Brie and Blueberry Chutney – A cup of honey, orange, and cinnamon Dinner: – 5 oz Chicken Nuggets With Mustard Honey Sauce – ½ oz of roasted potato sticks – Cabbage and carrot salad
Thursday	Breakfast: – 1 or 2 breakfast burritos – 1 glass of almond milk – 1 cup of fruit, cut into pieces (any flavor, except citrus fruits) Snack: – 1 slice of coconut bread – 1 cup of ginger or cinnamon tea or green tea Lunch: – 4½ oz baked pork chop – 5 oz Caesar salad – 4½ oz sautéed potatoes Afternoon snack: – A portion of Fig and Goat Cheese Crostini – 1 cup of green tea Dinner: – 5 oz cold veggie pizza sandwiches – 1 glass of natural juice
Friday	Breakfast: – 2 stuffed eggs

	– ½ cup of bread – 1 glass of papaya juice *Snack:* – 1 apple muffins – 1 cup of tea or coffee *Lunch:* – 5 oz of chicken in wine sauce – 9 oz of cranberry and almond celery logs – 1 glass of juice *Afternoon snack:* – A serving of Brie and Blueberry Chutney – A cup of ginger tea *Dinner:* – 5 oz Grilled Buttermilk Garlic Marinated Chicken – 1 cup of carrot, beet, and coriander salad
Saturday	*Breakfast:* – 1 bowl of Acai Berry Smoothie – 1 glass of homemade almond milk *Snack:* – 1/2 cup apple, cinnamon, and maple granola *Lunch:* – Chicken, pepper, and bacon wraps – 3 corn balls with cheese – 2 spring rolls of fresh tofu – 1 glass of natural juice or a glass of water flavored with cucumber and lemon *Afternoon snack:* – 2 slices of apple cinnamon bread – 1 cup of green tea or ginger or cinnamon *Dinner:* – 5 oz of Fig and Goat Cheese Crostini – 1 glass of natural juice
Sunday	*Breakfast:* – Dilly Scrambled Eggs – 2 layers of apple cinnamon French toast – 1 glass of natural juice *Snack:* – 1 slice of coconut bread – Ginger tea, cinnamon, mint *Lunch:* – 5 oz of Easy Turkey Sloppy Joes – 5 oz of Low Protein Baked Beef Tibbs Broccoli – 1 glass of natural juice *Afternoon snack:* – 1 Angelina's Gingerbread Muffins – 1 cup of tea *Dinner:* – 2 flour tortillas – 5 oz of bean dip – 1 glass of beet juice with apple

In addition to this eating plan, it is important to maintain fluid consumption. For this, we recommend drinking 4–6 glasses a day of cucumber water with lemon. Likewise, drink a glass of green juice on an empty stomach or at night before going to bed.

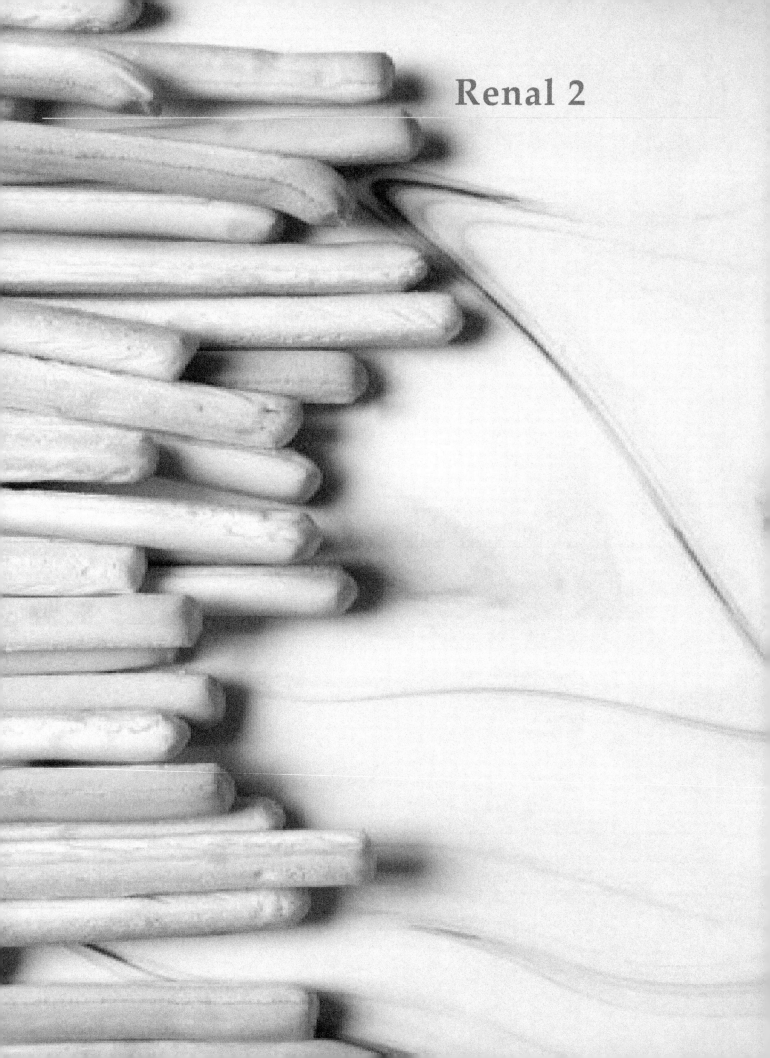

INTRODUCTION

Complying with a diet to prevent chronic diseases in our organism requires an individual commitment. Being aware of what to eat and what not to eat is fundamental to follow a diet plan. This does not prevent you from having to limit yourself to eating certain foods, the intention is that you can acquire the necessary knowledge to determine the portions you should consume.

To the extent that you comply with a balanced diet program as a healthy lifestyle, you can prevent not only kidney disease but also other conditions, the most common being diabetes and cardiovascular conditions.

Weight loss in combination with increased physical exercise can reduce the risks known as "metabolic syndrome." An individual with metabolic syndrome has three or more of these qualities:

- Fat stored around the abdomen
- High triglyceride levels in the blood
- Low levels of good cholesterol or HDL
- Low blood pressure
- High blood glucose levels
- Kidney failure

In this book, we want to provide you with a practical guide to an adequate food plan to keep the body in good working order. In the case of kidney disease, the patient must be clear about which foods should be consumed more regularly and which are less recommended.

Among the foods most recommended by nutrition professionals are:

1. **Natural foods:** since it means knowing their exact composition and estimating the loss of any citric compound, including potassium, after handling.
2. **Frozen foods:** studies have determined that the process of freezing and preservation of food helps to eliminate potassium.
3. **Vegetable foods:** are a viable alternative to avoid kidney diseases, since they do not usually have phosphates as preservatives. However, they should be washed well before consumption.

Another recommendation to optimize an eating plan is:

- Limit consumption of pre-cooked foods, as they usually have high preservative compounds, such as: sodium, phosphorus, among others.
- To prevent renal diseases, salt consumption should be limited. Instead, spices and flavoring herbs such as: chives, oregano, basil, bay leaf, juniper, rosemary, thyme, paprika, turmeric, etc., can be added.
- A lot of liquid should be consumed. It is essential to keep the body hydrated.
- Avoid consumption of saturated fats. Of all that we consume, fat is the most harmful to our health, since it contains twice as many calories as the same amount of sugar, starch or protein. Generally speaking, small amounts of foods high in fat are usually also high in calories.
  For example, ¼ cup of peanuts equals 19 gr. of fat and 215 gr. of calories; while 3 cups of peanuts for popcorns equals 0 gr. of fat and 60 gr. of calories.

Fat and diseases of the cardiovascular system and diabetes

Studies have shown that eating a high-fat diet increases cholesterol levels. Cholesterol is a type of fat in the blood, therefore, the higher the levels, the higher the probability of a heart attack and diabetes.

For this reason, it is essential to maintain a dietary program following the weight, fat and calorie goals required, as appropriate. Below is a table explaining the ideal daily fat and calorie intake of a person, according to his or her weight:

Weight (Kg.)	Fats (gr)	Calories
54-79	33	1.200
80-99	42	1.500
100-114	50	1.800
>150	55	2.000

Ways to eat foods with less fat and calories

1. **Eat less high-fat and high-calorie foods:** in these cases, the idea is to eat them at least once a week.
2. **Eat smaller amounts of high-fat and high-calorie foods:** to give you an example: to dress a bowl of salad, use a portion equivalent to 10 grams instead of using a ladle of dressing that equals approximately 32 grams.
3. **Consume more low-fat and low-calorie foods:** among these foods are: fruits, vegetables, vegetables, yogurt, whole grains, skim milk, low-fat cheeses, lean meats (without fat).
4. **Consume more omega-3 fatty acids:** it has been proven that this type of unsaturated fat can contribute to the proper functioning of the heart, helping to prevent diseases. Omega 3 fatty acids are present in certain fish, such as salmon, tuna, trout and sardines.
   They are also present in walnuts, flaxseed, flaxseed oil and canola oil. In this case, the American Heart Association recommends eating fish (85 to 120 grams per serving) at least twice a week.
5. **Learn to balance the calories you consume:** calories represent the energy level of food and beverages. Therefore, the number of calories in food will depend directly on the number of fats, carbohydrates, proteins and alcohol it contains.
6. **The balance of a good diet plan:** to prevent diseases and lose weight, the idea is to have a diet equivalent to 1200 calories in order to obtain a healthy and balanced diet. To prevent obesity, it is essential to control your diet and be more physically active.

Even though this book is focused on the Diet Plan for people with kidney problems, it is important to be able to distinguish the foods that contribute to a healthy organism and to the prevention of diseases, not only of the circulatory system but also of diabetes or the cardiovascular system.

It is important to emphasize that in the case of people with kidney problems, they should have the supervision of a nutrition specialist or the attending physician to follow up the diet plan.

On the other hand, the person must also be committed to daily physical activity of at least 30 minutes. Remember, the success of an eating plan for disease prevention must be combined with a daily exercise routine, as an elemental formula for a healthy body and mind.

95. GELATIN ENERGY CUBES WITH HIGH PROTEIN CONTENT

Servings: 3
Ingredients:
complementary
2 cups of water
3 small boxes of unsweetened strawberry jelly
2-1 / 4 cup cold water
1 box Knox® Original unflavored gelatin (4 sachets)
1-2 / 3 cups whey protein, strawberry flavor
Directions:
In a Pyrex measuring cup, microwave 2 cups of tap water to a boil.
Remove from microwave and slowly add the unsweetened gelatin to the boiling water while stirring continuously. Stir until powder is completely dissolved. Pour into a bowl.
In a mixing bowl, add 2-1/4 cups cold water, whey protein and unflavored gelatin powder. Stir well until no lumps or particles remain.
Slowly add the contents of the shaker to the strawberry gelatin mixture. Stir while adding.
Pour into a 9 "x 13" pan. Cover and refrigerate until firm. Cut into 48 cubes and divide into 8 equal portions.

Nutritional value:
- Energy value: 153 Kcal
- Protein: 7 g
- Carbohydrates: 16 g
- Fiber: 7 g
- Sugar: 5 g
- Sodium: 2 g
- Fat: 13 g
- Of which:
- - Saturated: 4 g
- - Monounsaturated: 6 g
- - Polyunsaturated: 2 g
- - Cholesterol: 115 mg

96. JELL-O CUBES RICH IN PROTEIN

Servings: 3
Ingredients:
1 small box of JELL-O, regular or unsweetened, any flavor
1/2 cup boiling water
1/2 cup cold water
1/2 cup whey protein powder
1/2 cup whipping cream
Directions:
Dissolve JELL-O in boiling water. Add cold water.
Whisk in protein powder until dissolved.
Place JELL-O in the refrigerator to set, approximately 30 minutes.

Cut into cubes and divide into 4 portions. Add a dollop of whipped cream and serve.

Nutritional value:
- Energy value: 78 Kcal
- Protein: 3 g
- Carbohydrates: 11 g
- Fiber: 3 g
- Sugar: 3 g
- Sodium: 1 g
- Fat: 8 g
- Of which:
- - Saturated: 4 g
- - Monounsaturated: 1 g
- - Polyunsaturated: 2 g
- - Cholesterol: 78 mg

97. HIGH-PROTEIN GELATIN CUPS

Servings: 2
Ingredients:
1 small box of gelatin, any flavor, regular or unsweetened.
3/4 cup boiling water
1 cup whey protein powder
3/4 cup cold water
Directions:
Dissolve the gelatin in the boiling water.
Dissolve the protein powder in the cold water.
After protein powder is completely dissolved, combine gelatin mixture with protein powder mixture.
Pour into 2-ounce soufflé cups and refrigerate until gelatinous.

Nutritional value:
- Energy value: 260 Kcal
- Protein: 5 g
- Carbohydrates: 16 g
- Fiber: 4 g
- Sugar: 4 g
- Sodium: 5 g
- Fat: 18 g
- Of which:
- - Saturated: 5 g
- - Monounsaturated: 7 g
- - Polyunsaturated: 4 g
- - Cholesterol: 119 mg

98. MULTICEREAL HOT CEREAL

Servings: 2
Ingredients:
1¾ cups of water.
2 tablespoons old-fashioned semolina, uncooked
1 tablespoon bulgur, uncooked
1 tablespoon whole buckwheat, toasted, uncooked
1 tablespoon oatmeal reduction oats, uncooked
3 tablespoons plain couscous, uncooked
Directions:
Bring water to a boil in a half-quart saucepan.
Add grits; stir shortly.
Add bulgur, buckwheat and oats; stir in shortly.
Reduce heat to a lively boil; spray generously with nonstick cooking spray over simmering surface.

Cover pot; simmer for 25 minutes.
Remove pot from heat; stir in couscous.
Let pot stand, covered, for 8 minutes, then serve.

Nutritional value:
- Energy value: 192 Kcal
- Protein: 19 g
- Carbohydrates: 15 g
- Fiber: 7 g
- Sugar: 3 g
- Sodium: 3 g
- Fat: 10 g
- Of which:
- - Saturated: 5 g
- - Monounsaturated: 3 g
- - Polyunsaturated: 1 g
- - Cholesterol: 127 mg

99. MAPLE AND HONEY NUT MIXTURE

Servings: 5
Ingredients:
3 cups Golden Grahams cereal
5 cups Rice Chex cereal
10 ounces of Teddy Grahams cinnamon snack crackers
6 ounces of pretzel crisps
1/2 cup unsalted butter
1/3 cup brown sugar
1/4 cup honey
1/4 cup maple syrup
5 ounces dried cranberries, sweetened
3 ounces Crispy Granny Smith apple chips
Directions:
Combine Golden Grahams, Rice Chex, Teddy Grahams and pretzels in a large bowl.
Melt butter in a small saucepan; add brown sugar, honey and maple syrup. Cook over low heat until sugar melts.
Pour over the cereal mixture and mix well until all pieces are coated.
Preheat oven to 325°F.
Prepare 3 jelly roll pans by lining with aluminum foil and spraying with cooking spray. (This can be done in 3 batches). Spread the cereal mixture evenly over the molds. Bake at 325°F for 20 minutes; however, stirring once halfway through.
Mix blueberries and apple chips; divide evenly among molds and stir. Bake 5 minutes longer; cool completely and store in an airtight container.

Nutritional value:
- Energy value: 153 Kcal
- Protein: 7 g
- Carbohydrates: 16 g
- Fiber: 7 g
- Sugar: 5 g
- Sodium: 2 g
- Fat: 13 g
- Of which:
- - Saturated: 4 g
- - Monounsaturated: 6 g
- - Polyunsaturated: 2 g
- - Cholesterol: 115 mg

100. GERMAN PANCAKES

Servings: 2
Ingredients:
2/3 cup all-purpose flour
2 tablespoons sugar

4 large eggs
1 cup of 1% skim milk
1/4 teaspoon vanilla extract
Directions:
In a medium bowl, integrate the flour and sugar. Add eggs and mix well with a whisk.
Add the milk and vanilla extract. Beat until clean.
Pour 3 tablespoons of the batter into a heated 8" or 10" nonstick skillet sprayed with nonstick cooking spray. Tilt the pan quickly to spread the batter. Cook until pancake is golden brown on the bottom (about forty-five seconds; edges will begin to dry out). Flip the pancake and brown the opposite side. Continue until all the batter is used.
Fold or roll thin cakes and serve with unfolded fruit, jam or syrup. If you prefer, add 1 to 2 tablespoons of ricotta or cream cheese for the filling.

Nutritional value:
- Energy value: 175 Kcal
- Protein: 13 g
- Carbohydrates: 11 g
- Fiber: 3 g
- Sugar: 2 g
- Sodium: 3 g
- Fat: 11 g
- Of which:
- - Saturated: 3 g
- - Monounsaturated: 5 g
- - Polyunsaturated: 2 g
- - Cholesterol: 87 mg

101. OATMEAL AND BLUEBERRY BREAKFAST COOKIES

Servings: 3
Ingredients:
1/2 cup unsalted butter
1/2 cup granulated sugar
1 large egg
1/4 cup whole wheat flour
1 teaspoon vanilla extract
Half teaspoon cinnamon
1/4 teaspoon salt
1.5 oz vanilla whey protein powder
1 cup applesauce
Three cups of rolled oats
One-half cup dried cranberries
Directions:
Set butter to melt at room temperature. Preheat oven to 350°F. Line a baking sheet with parchment paper.
With an electric mixer, mix the butter and sugar. Add the egg, flour, protein powder, vanilla extract, cinnamon and salt. Stir to combine.
Add into applesauce and integrate. Fold into the oats and cranberries.
Drop 1/4 cup spoonful of the cookie dough onto the baking sheet. Flatten each cookie just slightly.
Bake for 12 to 15 minutes, until cookies are golden brown but soft.
Let the cookies cool for five minutes on the baking sheet before transferring them to a wire rack to cool completely.

Nutritional value:
- Energy value: 260 Kcal
- Protein: 5 g
- Carbohydrates: 16 g
- Fiber: 4 g
- Sugar: 4 g
- Sodium: 5 g
- Fat: 18 g
- Of which:

- - Saturated: 5 g
- - Monounsaturated: 7 g
- - Polyunsaturated: 4 g
- - Cholesterol: 119 mg

102. EXCELLENT WAY TO START THE DAY BAGEL

Servings: 2
Ingredients:
1 bagel, 2 oz. size
2 tablespoons cream cheese
2 1/4-inch thick tomato slices
2 slices red onion
1 teaspoon low-sodium lemon pepper seasoning
Directions:
Slice bagel and toast until golden brown.
Spread cream cheese on each bagel half. Place onion slice and tomato ice if on top and sprinkle with lemon pepper seasoning.

Nutritional value:
- Energy value: 192 Kcal
- Protein: 19 g
- Carbohydrates: 15 g
- Fiber: 7 g
- Sugar: 3 g
- Sodium: 3 g
- Fat: 10 g
- Of which:
- - Saturated: 5 g
- - Monounsaturated: 3 g
- - Polyunsaturated: 1 g
- - Cholesterol: 127 mg

103. NO-BAKE OATMEAL PEANUT BARS

Servings: 2
Ingredients:
2 cups oat flakes, dry.
1/2 teaspoon cinnamon
1/8 teaspoon salt
1/2 cup whey protein powder
Half cup peanut butter
1/3 cup agave nectar
1/4 cup mini chocolate chips
Directions:
Line a five x 7-inch or eight-inch rectangular baking dish with waxed or parchment paper.
In a medium bowl, collectively mix together the oats, cinnamon and salt.
In a medium bowl, mix protein powder, peanut butter, and agave nectar; stir till clean.
Mix oats with peanut butter combination until well blended.
Spoon the combination lightly into a covered baking dish. Sprinkle chocolate chips on top and pat in lightly. Refrigerate for at least one hour.
Cut into five sections and then in half for 10 bars. If desired, wrap each bar in plastic wrap. Keep refrigerated until ready to eat or continue.

Nutritional value:
- Energy value: 185 Kcal
- Protein: 9 g
- Carbohydrates: 15 g
- Fiber: 7 g
- Sugar: 3 g
- Sodium: 3 g
- Fat: 10 g
- Of which:
- - Saturated: 5 g
- - Monounsaturated: 3 g
- - Polyunsaturated: 1 g
- - Cholesterol: 110 mg

104. FESTIVE MORNING FRENCH TOAST

Servings: 3
Ingredients:
3/4 cup brown sugar
1/2 cup unsalted butter
3 teaspoons cinnamon
3 large tart apples
1/2 cup sweetened, dried cranberries
1 pound Italian bread
6 large eggs
1-1 / 2 cups rice milk, not enriched
1 tablespoon vanilla
Directions:
Peel, core and thinly slice or chop apples.
In a thirteen "x 9" baking dish, combine brown sugar, melted butter and 1 teaspoon cinnamon. Add apples and cranberries; toss well to coat.
Spread the apple combination lightly over the bottom of the baking dish.
Cut bread into 3/4" slices and place on top of apple pinnacle.
Mix eggs, rice milk, vanilla and last 2 teaspoons cinnamon until well blended. Pour the aggregate over the bread, soaking the bread completely. Cover and refrigerate for four to 24 hours.
Preheat oven to 375° F.
Bake protected with aluminum foil for 30 minutes. Uncover the dish and bake for 15 minutes or until the pinnacle begins to brown.
Remove dish from oven and let stand for 5 minutes before cutting into 9 portions.
Serve hot. Dust the pinnacle with powdered sugar before serving.

Nutritional value:
- Energy value: 175 Kcal
- Protein: 13 g
- Carbohydrates: 11 g
- Fiber: 3 g
- Sugar: 2 g
- Sodium: 3 g
- Fat: 11 g
- Of which:
- - Saturated: 3 g
- - Monounsaturated: 5 g
- - Polyunsaturated: 2 g
- - Cholesterol: 87 mg

Brunch:

105. ONION AND HERB CRACKER FLATBREAD WITH PEACH SAUCE

Servings: 2

Ingredients:
1/2 cup Greek yogurt (fat-free)
3 tablespoons peach jam or preserves
1 tablespoon yellow mustard
1-3/4 cup white all-purpose flour
Mrs. Dash® herb and onion seasoning mix, 1 1/2 tablespoons
Sugar (two teaspoons)
1 cup water
1/3 cup of extra virgin olive oil
1 beaten egg white

Directions:
Combine yogurt or sour cream, peach jam and mustard in a small bowl. Place in refrigerator until ready to serve.
Preheat oven to 400°F.
Combine flour, Mrs. Dash seasoning and sugar in a medium bowl. In the middle of the Ingredients: dry, make a well. Combine water, oil and egg white in a bowl. Combine all Ingredients in a mixing bowl until a dough forms.
Knead the dough for 3-4 minutes on a floured board. Divide the dough into four equal parts and roll each into a ball.
Roll out the dough ball on a lightly floured board until very thin. Place on an ungreased baking sheet and cut into cookie slices or strips. To prevent the dough from bubbling, prick with a fork.
Bake for 7 to 9 minutes or until the croquettes are golden brown and crispy. Be careful not to overcook the food.
To make 4 dozen crackers, repeat with each dough ball.
Serve with Peachy Dip and crackers.

Nutritional value:
- Energy value: 227 Kcal
- Protein: 5 g
- Carbohydrates: 7 g
- Fiber: 5 g
- Sugar: 3 g
- Sodium: 2 g
- Fat: 9 g
- Of which:
- - Saturated: 7 g
- - Monounsaturated: 1 g
- - Polyunsaturated: 1 g
- Cholesterol: 100 mg

106. CELESTIAL JALÁ

Servings: 4

Ingredients:
7 cups whole wheat flour
2 tablespoons of baker's dry yeast
6 tablespoons of sugar
2 half cups of warm water
Half cup vegetable oil
2 teaspoons salt
1 large egg

Directions:
Place flour, yeast, sugar, water and oil in a large bowl and mix collectively. Knead the dough. When it forms a ball, add the salt.

Place the dough on a floured surface and keep kneading for 10 minutes, until the dough is clean and smooth and now not sticking. Coat the bowl and dough with 1 or two teaspoons of oil. Cover the bowl and place it in a warm area until the dough doubles in quantity (1 to 2 hours).
Knead the leavened dough for a couple of minutes. Divide the dough into 12 portions and roll each piece into a strand to be braided, about 10" to 12" at a time.
Braid 3 of the rolled dough strips collectively to form the challah.
Repeat with the last few strips of dough to make 4 challahs.
Place the challahs on a baking sheet or baking sheet, cover and let the dough push up once more, about 40 minutes.
Preheat oven to 350°F. Brush each Jala with beaten egg. Bake for about half an hour, until the jalás are golden brown. Remove the jalás from the oven and baking pan and cool on a wire rack.

Nutritional value:
- Energy value: 192 Kcal
- Protein: 19 g
- Carbohydrates: 15 g
- Fiber: 7 g
- Sugar: 3 g
- Sodium: 3 g
- Fat: 10 g
- Of which:
- - Saturated: 5 g
- - Monounsaturated: 3 g
- - Polyunsaturated: 1 g
- - Cholesterol: 127 mg

107. SAUSAGE AND EGG BREAKFAST SANDWICH

Servings: 1

Ingredients:
Non-stick spray oil
1/4 cup low-cholesterol liquid egg alternative LDL
1 English muffin
1 turkey sausage patty
1 tablespoon shredded natural cheddar cheese

Directions:
In a small skillet sprayed with nonstick cooking spray, pour egg product and prepare dinner over medium-low heat. When the egg appears to be almost cooked, flip it over with a spatula and cook 30 seconds longer.
Toast English muffin.
Place turkey sausage patty on a plate, cover with a paper towel and microwave dinner for 1 minute or the time indicated on the package. Assemble boiled egg on English muffin (fold to fit muffin). Top with sausage patty, then sharp cheddar cheese and last muffin 1/2.

Nutritional value:
- Energy value: 172 Kcal
- Protein: 13 g
- Carbohydrates: 12 g
- Fiber: 7 g
- Sugar: 3 g
- Sodium: 3 g
- Fat: 10 g
- Of which:
- - Saturated: 5 g
- - Monounsaturated: 3 g

- • - Polyunsaturated: 1 g
- • - Cholesterol: 120 mg

108. FESTIVE SCRAMBLED EGGS

Servings: 2
Ingredients:
3 halves cups low LDL liquid egg substitute
1/2 cup onion
1/2 cup pink bell pepper
Half cup green bell pepper
1 teaspoon black pepper
2 tablespoons trans-fat-free margarine
Directions:
Finely chop the onion and bell peppers.
Combine egg product, onion, bell peppers and black pepper in a bowl.

Melt margarine in a skillet. Add egg mixture and cook dinner until eggs are set. Stir frequently to prevent sticking.
Serve hot or place in warmer until ready to serve.

Nutritional value:
- • Energy value: 190 Kcal
- • Protein: 18 g
- • Carbohydrates: 14 g
- • Fiber: 7 g
- • Sugar: 3 g
- • Sodium: 3 g
- • Fat: 11g
- • Of which:
- • - Saturated: 5 g
- • - Monounsaturated: 3 g
- • - Polyunsaturated: 1 g
- • - Cholesterol: 120 mg

SIDE DISHES AND snacks:

109. PEANUT BUTTER AND CELERY JELLY LOGS

Servings: 2
Ingredients:
4 ribs of celery (medium, 8 inches)
4 tablespoons peanut butter (creamy)
2 tablespoons gelatin
Directions:
Trim ends of celery ribs.
1 tablespoon peanut butter, stuff into each celery rib.
On top of the peanut butter, spread the gelatin.
Serve each celery rib in three pieces.

Nutritional value:
- Energy value: 227 Kcal
- Protein: 5 g
- Carbohydrates: 7 g
- Fiber: 5 g
- Sugar: 3 g
- Sodium: 2 g
- Fat: 9 g
- Of which:
- - Saturated: 7 g
- - Monounsaturated: 1 g
- - Polyunsaturated: 1 g
- - Cholesterol: 100 mg

110. CREAM CHEESE COOKIES WITH FINGERPRINT

Servings: 4
Ingredients:
1 cup unsalted butter
8 oz cream cheese
2 cups flour for all motifs
2 tablespoons granulated sugar
2 teaspoons baking powder
1 teaspoon vanilla extract
Half cup strawberry jam
2 tablespoons powdered sugar
Directions:
Preheat oven to 350° F. Place butter and cream cheese to melt.
In a medium bowl combine flour, sugar and baking powder.
In a large bowl, incorporate butter, cream cheese and vanilla; beat until light and fluffy.
Add dry ingredients to the cream cheese addition and mix well. Form dough into a ball, wrap and chill for two hours.
Roll the dough to a thickness of one/four" on a lightly floured floor.
Cut with a 1 half inch spherical or fluted cutter.
Place 2" aside on an ungreased baking sheet. Press the center of each cookie lightly with your thumb and fill the center with 1/4 teaspoon of jam.
Bake for 10 to 12 minutes.
Remove from cookie sheet and place on a cooling rack.
Sift powdered sugar over the top of the cookie, if desired.

Nutritional value:
- Energy value: 175 Kcal
- Protein: 13 g
- Carbohydrates: 11 g
- Fiber: 3 g
- Sugar: 2 g
- Sodium: 3 g

- Fat: 11 g
- Of which:
- - Saturated: 3 g
- - Monounsaturated: 5 g
- - Polyunsaturated: 2 g
- - Cholesterol: 87 mg

111. EGG POCKETS

Servings: 2
Ingredients:
1¼ teaspoons dry yeast.
1 cup of warm water
1 tablespoon oil
1 tablespoon sugar
1 teaspoon garlic powder
2 cups all-purpose white flour
3/4 cup low LDL liquid egg substitute
4 tablespoons cream cheese
Butter flavored cooking spray
Directions:
Dissolve yeast in warm water.
Stir in oil, sugar, garlic powder and flour to make a smooth batter.
Place in a greased bowl, cover and set aside. Let relax for five minutes.
Roll out dough to 1/2-inch thickness. Cut into 4 pieces.
Scramble eggs and stir in cream cheese.
Place egg addition on half of each piece of dough. Fold the dough over, pinching the edges; then cut the pinnacle to vent.
Spray the top of each pocket with butter-flavored cooking spray.
Bake at 350°F for 15 to 20 minutes, until lightly browned.

Nutritional value:
- Energy value: 192 Kcal
- Protein: 19 g
- Carbohydrates: 15 g
- Fiber: 7 g
- Sugar: 3 g
- Sodium: 3 g
- Fat: 10 g
- Of which:
- - Saturated: 5 g
- - Monounsaturated: 3 g
- - Polyunsaturated: 1 g
- - Cholesterol: 127 mg

112. EGG IN A HOLE

Servings: 2
Ingredients:
1 massive egg
1 slice of bread
1/4 teaspoon Mrs. Dash Lemon Pepper seasoning combo
1 teaspoon grated Parmesan cheese
1 medium strawberry
Directions:
Use a cracker or cookie cutter to cut down the center of the bread slice to toast.
Spray each side of the bread and the center cut-out circle with cooking spray.

Heat a medium skillet and sear both pieces of the cut bread in the skillet. Crack the egg into the "hollow" center of the cut-out portion. Season with lemon pepper.

Cook for 1 to two minutes and flip to cook dinner on the other side. Additionally, flip the reduced bread circle to toast on all sides.

Sprinkle the egg with Parmesan cheese.

Serve egg and toast with a garnish of fresh strawberries.

Nutritional value:
- Energy value: 154Kcal
- Protein: 19 g
- Carbohydrates: 14 g
- Fiber: 7 g
- Sugar: 3 g
- Sodium: 3 g
- Fat: 11 g
- Of which:
- - Saturated: 5 g
- - Monounsaturated: 3 g
- - Polyunsaturated: 1 g
- - Cholesterol: 115 mg

113. AMAPOLA KRUNCH

Servings: 1
Ingredients:
12 cups unsalted popcorn.
1 and a third cups of sugar
1/2 cup corn syrup (light)
1 pound butter
1 teaspoon vanilla extract
Directions:
In a shallow pan, spread out the popcorn.
In a 1/2 quart saucepan, combine sugar, corn syrup and butter.
Cook over medium heat, stirring occasionally, until a small amount in cold water separates into thin strands that are hard but not brittle (a candy thermometer reading of 280°F). Remove the pan from the sun.
Pour in vanilla extract.
Pour the syrup over the popcorn and stir until evenly coated. Place on a greased baking sheet to cool. Cut into small pieces.
Allow time to cool. Refrigerate until ready to serve in an airtight container.

Nutritional value:
- Energy value: 153 Kcal
- Protein: 7 g
- Carbohydrates: 16 g
- Fiber: 7 g
- Sugar: 5 g
- Sodium: 2 g
- Fat: 13 g
- Of which:
- - Saturated: 4 g
- - Monounsaturated: 6 g
- - Polyunsaturated: 2 g
- - Cholesterol: 115 mg

114. FROZEN FRUIT DELIGHT

Servings: 4
Ingredients:
1/3 cup maraschino cherries
8 oz canned crushed pineapple
8 oz low-fat sour cream
1 tablespoon lemon juice
1 cup sliced strawberries
1/2 cup sugar
1/8 teaspoon salt
3 cups Reddi-Wip whipped topping

Directions:
Chop cherries and drain pineapple.
Place all ingredients except whipped topping, in a medium bowl and combine until well combined. Stir in whipped topping.
Place mixture in a freezable plastic field and freeze for 2 to three hours until hardened.

Nutritional value:
- Energy value: 227 Kcal
- Protein: 5 g
- Carbohydrates: 7 g
- Fiber: 5 g
- Sugar: 3 g
- Sodium: 2 g
- Fat: 9 g
- Of which:
- - Saturated: 7 g
- - Monounsaturated: 1 g
- - Polyunsaturated: 1 g
- - Cholesterol: 100 mg

115. POPCORN 3 WAYS

Servings: 1
Ingredients:
1/4 cup popcorn kernels (approximately)
1 teaspoon Sriracha hot chili sauce 1 1/2 tablespoons canola oil
4 tablespoons unsalted butter, melted
1/4 teaspoon nutritional yeast
2 teaspoon sugar (granulated)
Pinch of cinnamon
Directions:
In a medium saucepan, heat canola oil over medium-high heat.
Place three popcorn kernels in the pan and cover with a slightly cracked lid.
After the first three kernels have popped, add the remaining kernels to the pan and gently shake to coat with oil. Replace the slightly cracked lid back on the skillet.
The popcorn kernels will begin to pop quickly. Remove the skillet from the heat when it slowly pops and pour into three separate bowls.
In the first bowl, drizzle the chili sauce over the popcorn and toss gently to coat.
2 tablespoons nutritional yeast + 2 tablespoons melted butter Drizzle the remaining oil over the popcorn in the second bowl and toss gently to coat.
Combine cinnamon and sugar with remaining melted butter. Drizzle the remaining oil over the popcorn in the third bowl and toss gently to coat.
Each bowl should be divided into two servings, with one cup of each flavor of popcorn for each person.

Nutritional value:
- Energy value: 175 Kcal
- Protein: 13 g
- Carbohydrates: 11 g
- Fiber: 3 g
- Sugar: 2 g
- Sodium: 3 g
- Fat: 11 g
- Of which:
- - Saturated: 3 g
- - Monounsaturated: 5 g
- - Polyunsaturated: 2 g
- - Cholesterol: 87 mg

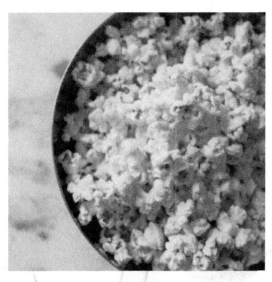

116.   POPCORN BALL

Servings: 4
Ingredients:
1 pound of butter
40 large marshmallows
Vanilla extract (1/2 teaspoon)
16 cups popcorn (unsalted)
1/2 teaspoon food coloring (red)
Directions:
In a saucepan, melt butter and marshmallows over low heat, stirring constantly. Remove from heat and stir in vanilla extract and food coloring, if desired.
In a large bowl, pour the popcorn. Stir in the marshmallow mixture. To make popcorn balls, grease your hands with butter and roll the popcorn into baseball-sized balls. Let cool on waxed paper. Wrap in plastic wrap, serve or store.

Nutritional value:
- Energy value: 67 Kcal
- Protein: 8 g
- Carbohydrates: 5 g
- Fiber: 5 g
- Sugar: 3 g
- Sodium: 2 g
- Fat: 15 g
- Of which:

- Saturated: 5 g
- Monounsaturated: 3 g
- Polyunsaturated: 6 g
- Cholesterol: 165 mg

117.   PICKLED OKRA

Servings: 4
Ingredients:
20 ounces frozen okra (optional)
2 tablespoons dill seeds
2 dried red peppers
2 whole chiles (canned)
4 cloves garlic
1 1/4 cups white vinegar
1 cup water
Directions:
Drain and thaw the okra.
Two-pint jars and lids should be sterilized.
1 teaspoon dill seeds, 1 teaspoon dill seeds, 1 teaspoon dill seeds, 1 teaspoon dill seeds, 1 teaspoon dill seeds, 1 teaspoon d Fill jars half full with okra.
1 red bell pepper, 1 chili bell pepper and 2 cloves of garlic in each jar.
Bring vinegar and water to a boil, then reduce to a simmer and cook for 5 minutes.
In each jar, pour the hot mixture over the okra. Close the jar and set it aside to cool.
Refrigerate for 2 weeks and the okra pickles will be ready to eat.

Nutritional value:
- Energy value: 227 Kcal
- Protein: 5 g
- Carbohydrates: 7 g
- Fiber: 5 g
- Sugar: 3 g
- Sodium: 2 g
- Fat: 9 g
- Of which:
- - Saturated: 7 g
- - Monounsaturated: 1 g
- - Polyunsaturated: 1 g
- Cholesterol: 100 mg

Vegetarian dishes:

118. CELERY STICKS WITH HUMMUS AND RED PEPPERS

Servings: 3
Ingredients: complementary
1 cup tomato sauce with roasted red peppers
1 cup onion
Three large eggs
3 pounds ground beef
1 cup raw oatmeal
6 tablespoons Parmesan cheese
1 tablespoon extra-virgin olive oil
1 teaspoon garlic powder
2 teaspoons oregano (dried)
1 teaspoon black pepper
Instructions
Prepare the tomato sauce with roasted red peppers (recipe from DaVita.com). Take it out of the equation.
Preheat oven to 375°F. Cut onion into small pieces.
In a large bowl, mix eggs, then add remaining Ingredients: and stir to combine.
Place 1" balls on a baking sheet.
Bake for 10 to 15 minutes or until meatballs are cooked through.
To serve, heat meatballs in a warming dish or slow cooker over low heat. 2 teaspoons sauce on the side or on the meatballs.

Nutritional value:
- Energy value: 227 Kcal
- Protein: 5 g
- Carbohydrates: 7 g
- Fiber: 5 g
- Sugar: 3 g
- Sodium: 2 g
- Fat: 9 g
- Of which:
- - Saturated: 7 g
- - Monounsaturated: 1 g
- - Polyunsaturated: 1 g
- - Cholesterol: 100 mg

119. PAKODA

Servings: 2
Ingredients:
1 medium onion
3 green chilies
Curry leaves, 2 teaspoons
Half teaspoon salt
A quarter teaspoon of baking soda
1 cup chickpea flour
1 pound rice flour
1 tablespoon margarine (trans fat-free)
1 teaspoon water
1 cup oil for frying
Directions:
Chop the onion, chilies and curry leaves into small pieces. Mix salt and baking soda well.
Combine chickpea flour, rice flour and melted margarine in a bowl.
Mix all ingredients (except oil) until smooth: (except oil) to a loose dough form, gradually adding small amounts of water as needed.
(Adjust as needed; you may need up to 2 tablespoons of water).

The oil should be hot. Small pieces of dough should be placed in the oil. Cook until golden brown and crisp.

Nutritional value:
- Energy value: 192 Kcal
- Protein: 19 g
- Carbohydrates: 15 g
- Fiber: 7 g
- Sugar: 3 g
- Sodium: 3 g
- Fat: 10 g
- Of which:
- - Saturated: 5 g
- - Monounsaturated: 3 g
- - Polyunsaturated: 1 g
- - Cholesterol: 127 mg

120. GRILLED CORN PANCAKES WITH CHEESE (AREPAS)

Servings: 2
Ingredients:
2/3 cup white corn flour
4 ounces of coastal cheese
Half teaspoon of aniseed
1 cup of warm water
1 teaspoon of butter
Directions:
Place the corn flour in a bowl.
Grate the cheese and add the cheese and anise to the flour.
Add the warm water; mix with a spatula.
Let stand for 10 minutes and then knead for 2 to 3 minutes.
To shape the corn puddings, make 4 circles about 4 inches wide and 1/2 inch thick.
Grease a skillet or arepa pan with butter. Place each corn cake in the skillet or arepa pan and cook until lightly browned.

Nutritional value:
- Energy value: 153 Kcal
- Protein: 7 g
- Carbohydrates: 16 g
- Fiber: 7 g
- Sugar: 5 g
- Sodium: 2 g
- Fat: 13 g
- Of which:
- - Saturated: 4 g
- - Monounsaturated: 6 g
- - Polyunsaturated: 2 g
- - Cholesterol: 115 mg

121. OMELETTE DE ESPAGUETI WITH ALBAHACA

Servings: 4
Ingredients:
1/3 cup green onion

2 tablespoons of sparkling basil
2 half cups of whole wheat spaghetti, cooked
1/3 cup 1% low-fat milk
4 large eggs
2 large egg whites
1/4 teaspoon black pepper
2 oz. Mozzarella cheese

Directions:

Chop inexperienced onion and basil; set aside.

Coat a medium nonstick skillet with 2 teaspoons olive oil. Spread the cooked spaghetti lightly in the skillet and prepare dinner over medium heat for 2 minutes.

Whisk milk, eggs, egg whites and black pepper collectively in a bowl. Pour gently over the pasta. Sprinkle the top of the frittata with cheese, green onions and basil. Cover and prepare dinner for about eight minutes till set.

Cut the frittata into four wedges and serve.

Nutritional value:
- Energy value: 175 Kcal
- Protein: 13 g
- Carbohydrates: 11 g
- Fiber: 3 g
- Sugar: 2 g
- Sodium: 3 g
- Fat: 11 g
- Of which:
- - Saturated: 3 g
- - Monounsaturated: 5 g
- - Polyunsaturated: 2 g
- - Cholesterol: 87 mg

122.   BLUEBERRY AND ROASTED GARLIC RISOTTO

Servings: 2

Ingredients:
1 cup onion
2 tablespoons butter
3 tablespoons roasted garlic
3/4 cup Arborio rice, uncooked
2 cups low sodium chicken broth
1/2 cup sweetened, dried cranberries
1/2 tablespoon Parmesan cheese

Directions:

Preheat oven to 425°F. Spray a pan with nonstick cooking spray.

Chop the onion.

Melt butter in a large saucepan. Add roasted garlic and onion to the saucepan and cook over medium heat until soft.

Add rice and cook for 2 minutes.

Add the broth and dried cranberries to the rice mixture. Bring to a boil and cook for 2 minutes.

Pour into casserole dish. Cover and bake for 30 minutes.

Remove from oven and sprinkle Parmesan cheese on top. Serve immediately.

Nutritional value:
- - Energy value: 175 Kcal
- - Protein: 13 g
- - Carbohydrates: 11 g
- - Fiber: 3 g
- - Sugar: 2 g
- - Sodium: 3 g
- - Fat: 11 g
- - Of which:
- - Saturated: 3 g
- - Monounsaturated: 5 g
- - Polyunsaturated: 2 g
- - Cholesterol: 87 mg

123.   PIEROGI WITH SWEET CABBAGE AND MUSHROOM FILLING

Servings: 4

Ingredients:
2 quarts of cabbage
1 pound of onion
1/2 pound mushrooms
1 cup all-purpose flour
One large egg
1 tablespoon trans-fat-free margarine
2 tablespoons hot water
1 tablespoon cooking oil
1/4 teaspoon freshly ground pepper

Directions:

The cabbage should be finely shredded, the onion should be finely chopped and the mushrooms should be thinly sliced.

Create a well in the center of the flour in a tub. Combine, e.g., g, melted margarine and hot water in a mixing bowl.

With a pastry knife, blend until a dough forms. Knead the dough on a board until smooth. Form into a ball, wrap in plastic wrap and let rest for one hour.

Fill a medium saucepan halfway with water and bring to a boil. Reduce the heat to low and cook for 15 to 20 minutes, or until the vegetables are tender. Drain and suck excess liquid from the cabbage.

Use 1 tablespoon oil to sauté chopped onions and mushrooms until lightly caramelized.

Combine cabbage, onion and mushrooms in a mixing bowl. Allow to cool before serving.

Finely chop the vegetable mixture once it has cooled. Add a pinch of pepper to taste.

Make a 10 "to 11" circle with the dough. Using a round cookie cutter, cut out 12 circles from the dough.

Fill each dough circle with a heaping teaspoon of filling. To make a crescent-shaped ball of dough, fold it over, roll it out and press the sides together.

Drop two or three dough balls at a time into a pot of boiling water. When the pierogi is finished, it will float to the tip. With a skimmer, remove the chicken.

If necessary, gently fry the dumplings in oil once they are boiled.

Nutritional value:
- Energy value: 192 Kcal
- Protein: 19 g
- Carbohydrates: 15 g
- Fiber: 7 g
- Sugar: 3 g
- Sodium: 3 g
- Fat: 10 g
- Of which:
- - Saturated: 5 g
- - Monounsaturated: 3 g
- - Polyunsaturated: 1 g
- - Cholesterol: 127 mg

124.   MUSHROOMS AND RED BELL PEPPER OMELET

Servings: 2

Ingredients:
1/2 cup of raw mushrooms portions
2 tablespoons onion
1/4 cup canned sweet crimson peppers

2 teaspoons butter
3 large eggs
1 teaspoon Worcestershire sauce
2 tablespoons whipped cream cheese
1/4 teaspoon black pepper

Directions:

Dice mushrooms, onion and crimson peppers.

Melt 1 teaspoon butter in a skillet over medium heat. Add mushrooms and onion; sauté five minutes until onion is soft. Add diced pink pepper. Remove vegetables from skillet and set aside.

Melt the last teaspoon of butter inside the skillet. Beat eggs with Worcestershire sauce and cook over medium heat. Cook the omelet calmly by shaking the pan and gently lifting the edges to allow the raw egg to run under the cooked egg.

When eggs are partially cooked, cover with vegetable topping. Place spoonfuls of whipped cream cheese on top of vegetables. Continue cooking until eggs are set.

Remove the skillet from heat and fold the omelet in half. Sprinkle with pepper. Divide into batches and serve.

Nutritional value:
- Energy value: 152 Kcal
- Protein: 18 g
- Carbohydrates: 15 g
- Fiber: 7 g
- Sugar: 3 g
- Sodium: 3 g
- Fat: 9 g
- Of which:
- - Saturated: 5 g
- - Monounsaturated: 3 g
- - Polyunsaturated: 1 g
- - Cholesterol: 120 mg

125. CREAMY ORZO AND VEGETABLES

Servings: 2

Ingredients:
1 clove of garlic
1 small onion
1 small zucchini
1 medium carrot
2 tablespoons olive oil
1 teaspoon curry powder
3 cups low sodium chicken broth
1/4 teaspoon salt
1 cup orzo pasta, uncooked
1/4 cup grated Parmesan cheese
2 tablespoons fresh parsley
1/2 cup frozen peas
1/4 teaspoon black pepper

Directions:

Finely chop the garlic. Chop the onion and zucchini. Shred the carrots.

In a large skillet, heat the olive oil over medium heat. Sauté garlic, onion, zucchini and carrots for 5 minutes.

Add curry powder, chicken broth and salt; bring to a boil.

Add the orzo pasta and stir until the mixture returns to a boil. Cover and reduce heat to a simmer. Cook, stirring occasionally for about 10 minutes until liquid is absorbed and pasta is al dente.

Stir in the cheese, chopped parsley and frozen peas. Heat until vegetables are hot, adding a little more broth if necessary to maintain creaminess. Add pepper to taste.

Nutritional value:
- Energy value: 175 Kcal
- Protein: 13 g
- Carbohydrates: 11 g

- Fiber: 3 g
- Sugar: 2 g
- Sodium: 3 g
- Fat: 11 g
- Of which:
- - Saturated: 3 g
- - Monounsaturated: 5 g
- - Polyunsaturated: 2 g
- - Cholesterol: 87 mg

126. RICE PILAF BETTER THAN PACKAGED

Servings: 2

Ingredients:
2 ounces noodles, uncooked
2 tablespoons unsalted butter
1 cup parboiled rice, uncooked
2 cups water
1 tablespoon onion-herb seasoning mix
1 teaspoon chicken-flavored bouillon granules

Directions:

In a skillet over medium heat, melt 1 tablespoon butter.

Break noodles into 2-inch pieces and cook, stirring frequently until noodles begin to brown.

Add remaining butter and rice. Stir to combine.

Add water, Mrs. Dash herb seasoning and chicken stock granules to the pan. Stir to combine ingredients.

Cover and bring to a boil. Reduce to a simmer and simmer for 20 minutes. Do not remove the lid.

Turn off heat and let stand covered for 5 more minutes.

Stir with a fork and serve.

Nutritional value:
- Energy value: 153 Kcal
- Protein: 7 g
- Carbohydrates: 16 g
- Fiber: 7 g
- Sugar: 5 g
- Sodium: 2 g
- Fat: 13 g
- Of which:
- - Saturated: 4 g
- - Monounsaturated: 6 g
- - Polyunsaturated: 2 g
- - Cholesterol: 115 mg

127. CARAWAY CABBAGE AND RICE

Servings: 2

Ingredients:
Non-stick spray oil
1 cup cabbage
1 tablespoon onion
1/4 cup water
1 tablespoon Worcestershire sauce
1/2 teaspoon caraway seeds
1/4 cup canned mandarin oranges
1 cup cooked rice

Directions:

Shred the cabbage and chop the onion.

Spray a nonstick skillet with cooking spray and sauté onion and cabbage until soft.

Add water, Worcestershire sauce and caraway seeds. Cook for 3 minutes. Stir to avoid burning.

Drain mandarin oranges and add to cabbage mixture. Add the hot rice.

Remove from heat and serve.

Nutritional value:
- Energy value: 192 Kcal
- Protein: 19 g
- Carbohydrates: 15 g
- Fiber: 7 g
- Sugar: 3 g
- Sodium: 3 g
- Fat: 10 g
- Of which:
- - Saturated: 5 g
- - Monounsaturated: 3 g
- - Polyunsaturated: 1 g
- Cholesterol: 127 mg

128. ELEGANT AND EASY LEMON RICE WITH VEGETABLES

Servings: 2

Ingredients:
1/2 cup celery
1/4 cup onion
1-1 / 2 cups fresh mushrooms
3 tablespoons unsalted margarine
1-1 / 4 cups water
1 teaspoon lemon zest
2 tablespoons lemon juice
1/8 teaspoon dried whole thyme
1/8 teaspoon black pepper
1/8 teaspoon original herb seasoning
10 tablespoons rice, uncooked

Directions:
Chop celery and mince onion. Thinly slice mushrooms.

Sauté celery and onion in 1-1/2 tablespoons margarine in a large skillet.

Stir in water, lemon zest, lemon juice, thyme, pepper and herb seasoning. Transfer to a bowl.

Add the rice, bring the water back to a boil, then cover, reduce the heat and simmer for 20 minutes until the rice is tender.

Melt the remaining 1-1/2 tablespoons margarine in a small skillet. Sauté mushrooms until tender.

Pour mushrooms into the rice mixture and stir to combine. Serve hot and enjoy.

Nutritional value:
- Energy value: 153 Kcal
- Protein: 7 g
- Carbohydrates: 16 g
- Fiber: 7 g
- Sugar: 5 g
- Sodium: 2 g
- Fat: 13 g
- Of which:
- - Saturated: 4 g
- - Monounsaturated: 6 g
- - Polyunsaturated: 2 g
- Cholesterol: 115 mg

FISHES:

129. CHRISTMAS TUNA FISH BALL

Servings: 2
Ingredients:
8 ounces cream cheese
5 ounces canned tuna
1/3 cup dried, sweetened cranberries
1/4 cup celery
2 tablespoons red onion
1/4 teaspoon ground cumin
1/4 cup dry unseasoned bread crumbs
1 tablespoon dried parsley
Directions:
Set cream cheese to soften for 30 minutes.
Drain canned tuna and flake with a fork.
In a bowl, combine cream cheese, tuna, blueberries, celery, onion and cumin. Mix with an electric mixer until well combined.
Combine the bread crumbs and parsley and then place on a plate.
Form the cream cheese mixture into a ball and roll in the breadcrumbs to coat.
Wrap the ball in plastic wrap and refrigerate until ready to serve.

Nutritional value:
• Energy value: 189 Kcal
• Protein: 19 g
• Carbohydrates: 15 g
• Fiber: 7 g
• Sugar: 5 g
• Sodium: 3 g
• Fat: 10 g
• Of which:
• - Saturated: 3 g
• - Mononounsaturated: 5 g
• - Polyunsaturated: 1 g
• - Cholesterol: 79 mg

130. CHRISTMAS CHEESE BALL

Servings: 2
Ingredients:
8 ounces cream cheese
1/4 cup Catalina or Russian salad dressing
1 teaspoon onion powder
1/3 cup finely ground walnuts
Directions:
Soften cream cheese.
In a medium bowl combine cream cheese, salad dressing and onion powder.
Place in the refrigerator for 30 minutes to chill.
Form cheese mixture into a ball.
Place the ground nuts on a plate and roll the cheese ball to coat.
Wrap the cheese ball in plastic wrap and chill until ready to serve.

Nutritional value:
• Energy value: 227 Kcal
• Protein: 5 g
• Carbohydrates: 7 g
• Fiber: 5 g
• Sugar: 3 g

• Sodium: 2 g
• Fat: 9 g
• Of which:
• - Saturated: 7 g
• - Mononounsaturated: 1 g
• - Polyunsaturated: 1 g
• - Cholesterol: 100 mg

131. CREAMY SHELLS WITH PEAS AND BACON

Servings: 2
Ingredients:
2 tablespoons unsalted butter
1 cup half-fat ricotta cheese
1/2 cup grated Parmesan cheese
1/4 teaspoon black pepper
3 slices of bacon, uncooked
1 tablespoon olive oil
1 cup onion
3 cloves garlic
1-1 / 2 cups small whole wheat shell pasta, uncooked
3/4 cup frozen peas
1 tablespoon lemon juice
Directions:
Bring 4 quarts of water to a boil in a large pot to cook the pasta.
Cut the butter into pieces. Place the ricotta, Parmesan cheese, butter and pepper in a bowl large enough to hold the pasta, when cooked.
Cut bacon into 1/4" strips. In a medium nonstick skillet over medium heat add the oil and bacon. Fry until crisp, 6 to 7 minutes. Transfer the bacon to a plate lined with paper towels.
Chop the onion and mince the garlic. Add the onion to the same skillet and cook until lightly browned, about 3 minutes. Add garlic and cook until fragrant, about 1 minute. Transfer the onion mixture to the bowl with the ricotta mixture.
Bring pasta to a boil. When the pasta is about 1 minute from al dente (still a little tough), add the peas and continue cooking for 1 minute. Reserve 1 cup of the cooking water, then drain the pasta and peas.
Add 1/2 cup of the reserved cooking water and the lemon juice to the ricotta mixture and whisk until smooth. Add the pasta and peas to the bowl and toss to coat, adding more of the reserved cooking water as needed to moisten the pasta. Stir in the crisp bacon and add additional pepper to taste.

Nutritional value:
• Energy value: 153 Kcal
• Protein: 7 g
• Carbohydrates: 16 g
• Fiber: 7 g
• Sugar: 5 g
• Sodium: 2 g
• Fat: 13 g
• Of which:
• - Saturated: 4 g
• - Mononounsaturated: 6 g
• - Polyunsaturated: 2 g
- Cholesterol: 115 mg

MEATS:

132. FANTASTIC PORK FAJITAS

Servings: 2
Ingredients:
1 green bell pepper
1 medium onion
2 garlic cloves
1 pound of lean and boneless pork meat
1 teaspoon dried oregano
Half teaspoon cumin
Pineapple juice (two tablespoons)
2 teaspoons apple cider vinegar
1/4 teaspoon cayenne pepper
1 tablespoon canola oil
4 flour tortillas, 8 corn tortillas "about the size.

Directions:
Green bell pepper and onion should be sliced. Garlic cloves should be minced. With a sharp knife, cut pork across the grain into 1/8-inch thick papery slices."

In a gallon-sized resealable plastic container, combine the garlic, oregano, pineapple juice, vinegar and hot sauce. Marinate pork for 10 to 15 minutes.

Preheat oven to 325°F. While the pork is cooking, wrap the tortillas in aluminum foil and heat them.

Heat a large skillet or griddle until very hot. Combine the fat, onion, green bell pepper and pork strips in a large mixing bowl. Stir-fry for about 5 minutes or until pork is no longer pink.

Serve with warm flour tortillas, divided into four parts.

Nutritional value:
- Energy value: 227 Kcal
- Protein: 5 g
- Carbohydrates: 7 g
- Fiber: 5 g
- Sugar: 3 g
- Sodium: 2 g
- Fat: 9 g
- Of which:
- - Saturated: 7 g
- - Monounsaturated: 1 g
- - Polyunsaturated: 1 g
- - Cholesterol: 100 mg

133. LUMPIA

Servings: 2
Ingredients:
2 cloves garlic
1/2 cup white onion
2 onions (green)
1 pound of pork field
1 tablespoon canola oil
1 cup coleslaw dressing
1 teaspoon ground black pepper
1 teaspoon garlic powder
1 teaspoon soy sauce (low sodium)
A total of 30 lumpia wraps
2 cups cooking (peanut) oil.

Directions:
Garlic should be minced. White and green onions should be chopped.

Brown ground pork in a large skillet. Remove pork from skillet and set aside to drain on paper towels.

Canola oil should be used to coat the pan. Sauté garlic and white onion until onion is translucent.

Continue cooking the coleslaw mixture, green onions and browned pork in the skillet. To combine, stir everything together.

Add the pepper, garlic powder and low sodium soy sauce to the mixture. Remove the skillet from the heat and set aside until cool enough to eat.

Place 2 tablespoons of the filling mixture diagonally near one corner of the lumpia wrapper, leaving space at both ends. Fold the near side over the filling, then fold both sides over and roll up tightly. To close the wrapper, moisten one edge with water.

Repeat with the rest of the wraps. To keep the rolls from drying out, wrap them in plastic wrap. Heat a deep skillet over medium heat and add 1/2 cup peanut oil, heating for 5 minutes. Carefully drop 3-4 lumpia into the liquid. Fry until golden brown, about 1 to 2 minutes. Using paper towels, absorb excess liquid. Serve immediately or wrap and reheat later.

Nutritional value:
- Energy value: 175 Kcal
- Protein: 13 g
- Carbohydrates: 11 g
- Fiber: 3 g
- Sugar: 2 g
- Sodium: 3 g
- Fat: 11 g
- Of which:
- - Saturated: 3 g
- - Monounsaturated: 5 g
- - Polyunsaturated: 2 g
- - Cholesterol: 87 mg

134. LEMONADE WINGS

Servings: 2
Ingredients:
1/4 cup onion
4 teaspoons rosemary (fresh)
1/4 cup canola oil
1 tablespoon butter
1 liter of lemonade
1/4 teaspoon black pepper
24 drummettes of chicken wings

Directions:
Preheat oven to 400°F.

Chop the onion and rosemary into small pieces.

In a baking dish, place the chicken wings.

In a saucepan, combine the remaining ingredients and cook for 3 minutes.

Bake for 30 to 35 minutes after pouring the mixture over the chicken. Check to see if anything is done.

Serve wings immediately or keep warm in a covered dish or crock pot until ready to eat.

Nutritional value:
- Energy value: 192 Kcal
- Protein: 19 g
- Carbohydrates: 15 g
- Fiber: 7 g
- Sugar: 3 g
- Sodium: 3 g
- Fat: 10 g
- Of which:
- - Saturated: 5 g
- - Monounsaturated: 3 g
- - Polyunsaturated: 1 g

- Cholesterol: 127 mg

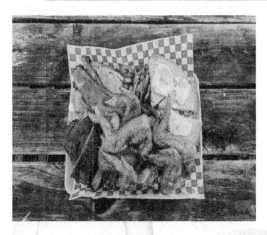

135. ITALIAN MEATBALLS

Servings: 4
Ingredients:
1 cup tomato sauce with roasted red peppers
1 onion (cup)
3 eggs (large)
3 pounds of beef (ground)
1 cup raw oatmeal
6 tablespoons Parmesan cheese, grated
1 tablespoon extra-virgin olive oil
1 tablespoon garlic powder
2 teaspoons dried oregano
1 teaspoon ground black pepper
Directions:
Prepare tomato sauce with roasted red peppers (recipe from DaVita.com). Eliminate from the equation.
Preheat oven to 375°F. Finely chop the onion.
In a large bowl, mix eggs, then add remaining Ingredients: and stir well.
Place on a baking sheet and roll into 1" balls.
Bake for 10 to 15 minutes or until meatballs are cooked through.
Place meatballs in a warming dish or slow cooker on low heat to serve. Serve meatballs with 2 teaspoons sauce on the side or in the meatballs.

Nutritional value:
- Energy value: 153 Kcal
- Protein: 7 g
- Carbohydrates: 16 g
- Fiber: 7 g
- Sugar: 5 g
- Sodium: 2 g
- Fat: 13 g
- Of which:
- - Saturated: 4 g
- - Monounsaturated: 6 g
- - Polyunsaturated: 2 g
- - Cholesterol: 115 mg

136. HULA DUMPLINGS

Servings: 1
Ingredients:
4 ribs of celery (medium, 8 inches).
Red bell pepper, 2 tablespoons.
Hummus (four tablespoons)
Directions:

Trim the ends of the celery ribs. Red peppers should be cut into 1/4-inch squares.
Using 1 tablespoon of hummus, fill each celery rib.
Each celery rib should be cut into three sections.
On each piece of celery filled with hummus, place 2 red bell pepper slices.

Nutritional value:
- Energy value: 175 Kcal
- Protein: 13 g
- Carbohydrates: 11 g
- Fiber: 3 g
- Sugar: 2 g
- Sodium: 3 g
- Fat: 11 g
- Of which:
- - Saturated: 3 g
- - Monounsaturated: 5 g
- - Polyunsaturated: 2 g
- - Cholesterol: 87 mg

137. STOVE CASSEROLE OF GROUND MEAT AND GREEN PEAS

Servings: 2
Ingredients:
3 cups of fresh potatoes
1 medium onion
1 lb. lean ground beef
2 1/2 cups liquid
3 cups fresh green peas, shelled
2 cups beef broth (low sodium)
Cornstarch (2 tablespoons)
Directions:
Place potatoes, peeled and cubed, in a large pot of water and bring to a boil. Remove the pan from the heat, drain the water and replace it with fresh water at room temperature. Cook for 10 minutes after boiling the potatoes. Drain the water.
Finely chop the onion. In a 3-quart skillet, cook ground beef, onion and 1/2 cup water until the meat is crumbled and browned.
Mix the ground beef mixture with the potatoes, peas and the remaining 2 cups of water. Simmer for another 10 minutes, or until tender.
1/4 cup beef broth + 1/4 cup cornstarch + 1/4 cup beef broth + 1/4 cup beef broth + 1/4 cup beef broth + 1/4 cup beef broth + 1/4 cup beef broth + 1/4 cup beef broth + 1/4 cup beef broth + 1/4
Simmer cornstarch mixture with remaining broth in skillet until casserole is thickened.
Serve immediately and enjoy!

Nutritional value:
- Energy value: 153 Kcal
- Protein: 7 g
- Carbohydrates: 16 g
- Fiber: 7 g
- Sugar: 5 g
- Sodium: 2 g
- Fat: 13 g
- Of which:
- - Saturated: 4 g
- - Monounsaturated: 6 g
- - Polyunsaturated: 2 g
- Cholesterol: 115 mg

EASY CHORIZO

Servings: 2
Ingredients:
3 cloves garlic
1 pound of 85 percent lean ground beef
2 tablespoons chili powder (hot)
2 tablespoons oil (canola)
Paprika (1 tablespoon)
White vinegar, 2 teaspoons
2 teaspoons cayenne or red bell pepper
1 teaspoon freshly ground black pepper
1 teaspoon oregano, powdered
Directions:
Garlic should be finely minced.
In a large bowl, combine all ingredients well. Refrigerate for 12 to 24 hours in an airtight jar.
Alternatively, divide the recipe into 1/4 cup sections and store all. Cover with plastic wrap or brown paper and freeze for later use in heavy plastic freezer bags.
Cook a 1/4 cup portion per person in a nonstick or greased skillet on the stove when ready to eat. Using a spatula, finely shred the meat. If necessary, use in DaVita.com's egg and chorizo omelet recipe.

Nutritional value:
- Energy value: 192 Kcal
- Protein: 19 g
- Carbohydrates: 15 g
- Fiber: 7 g
- Sugar: 3 g
- Sodium: 3 g
- Fat: 10 g
- Of which:
- - Saturated: 5 g
- - Monounsaturated: 3 g
- - Polyunsaturated: 1 g
- Cholesterol: 127 mg

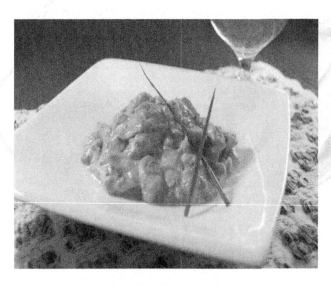

139. EASY VEAL STROGANOFF IN A CROCKPOT

Servings: 2
Ingredients:
1/2 cup onion
2 cloves garlic
1 pound boneless beef, cut into 1" cubes
1 cup beef broth (low sodium)
1/3 cup sherry (dry)

1/2 teaspoon dried oregano
1/4 teaspoon freshly ground black pepper
1/8 teaspoon dried thyme
1 bay leaf
1/2 cup sour cream
1/4 cup flour (all-purpose)
A couple of teaspoons of water
12 ounces uncooked egg noodles
Directions:
Finely chop onion and garlic cloves.
In a crockpot, combine the beef, broth, sherry, onion, garlic, oregano, pepper, thyme and bay leaf. Cover and cook over high heat for 4 to 5 hours, or until meat is tender.
Combine sour cream, flour and water in a bowl and mix until smooth.
Allow another 15 to 25 minutes for the sour cream mixture to thicken before applying it to the meat in the slow cooker.
Cook the egg noodles as directed on the box, omitting the salt. Drain the water.
Over the egg noodles, serve the stroganoff.

Nutritional value:
- Energy value: 175 Kcal
- Protein: 13 g
- Carbohydrates: 11 g
- Fiber: 3 g
- Sugar: 2 g
- Sodium: 3 g
- Fat: 11 g
- Of which:
- - Saturated: 3 g
- - Monounsaturated: 5 g
- - Polyunsaturated: 2 g
- - Cholesterol: 87 mg

140. INDIAN CHICKEN CURRY

Servings: 2
Ingredients:
1 medium tomato
2 medium onions
2 garlic cloves
1 ginger root in one-inch cubes
5 tablespoons vegetable oil
3/4 teaspoon whole cumin seeds
1 cinnamon stick
2 bay leaves
1/4 teaspoon peppercorns, whole
1/2 pound small chicken thighs
3/4 teaspoon salt
1-1 / 2 teaspoons cayenne pepper
1/2 teaspoon garam masala
Directions:
Peel and chop the tomato. Chop the onion, garlic and ginger root. Remove the skin from the chicken and discard.
Heat the oil in a large, wide pot over medium-high heat. When hot, place in the cumin seeds, cinnamon, bay leaves and peppercorns. Stir as soon as.
Add the onions, garlic and ginger. Stir this mixture till the onion alternatives form brown specks.
Add the tomatoes, hen, salt and cayenne pepper. Stir to combine and bring to a boil.
Cover the pot tightly, turn the heat to low and simmer for 25 minutes or until the chicken is tender. Stir a few times during this cooking time.
Remove the lid and raise the heat to medium. Sprinkle in the garam masala and cook, stirring gently for about five minutes to reduce the liquid.

Nutritional value:
- Energy value: 144 Kcal
- Protein: 19 g
- Carbohydrates: 9 g
- Fiber: 3 g
- Sugar: 1 g
- Sodium: 3 g
- Fat: 4 g
- Of which:
- - Saturated: 1 g
- - Monounsaturated: 2 g
- - Polyunsaturated: 1 g
- - Cholesterol: 73 mg

141. JAMAICAN CHICKEN

Servings: 2
Ingredients:
6 medium onions without experience
1 small onion
2 teaspoons fresh ginger
3 cloves garlic
2 habanero peppers or 1 scotch bonnet chili bell pepper
2 tablespoons white vinegar
1 tablespoon soy sauce
1 tablespoon canola oil
2 tablespoons brown sugar
1 teaspoon sea or kosher salt
2 teaspoons fresh thyme
1 teaspoon allspice
1/4 teaspoon black pepper
1/4 teaspoon nutmeg
1/8 teaspoon cinnamon
1-1 / 2 pounds boneless, skinless poultry drumsticks
Directions:
Coarsely chop the green and yellow onions. Peel and mince the ginger. Mince the garlic cloves. Sow and chop the hot peppers.
Place all ingredients, besides fowl, in a food processor and process until smooth.
Place chicken and combined combination on a plate or in a large zip-lock bag. Seal and refrigerate to marinate for 3 to 24 hours.
Remove the bird from the field and discard the last of the marinade. Heat a grill to medium-high heat. Grease the grill grate, then add the bird and cook dinner on each side for approximately 10 to 12 minutes. The chicken should reach one hundred sixty-five° F before discarding it from the grill.

Nutritional value:
- Energy value: 192 Kcal
- Protein: 19 g
- Carbohydrates: 15 g
- Fiber: 7 g
- Sugar: 3 g
- Sodium: 3 g
- Fat: 10 g
- Of which:
- - Saturated: 5 g
- - Monounsaturated: 3 g
- - Polyunsaturated: 1 g
- - Cholesterol: 127 mg

142. QUICK GLAZED CHICKEN

Servings: 1
Ingredients:
2 teaspoons olive oil
1 pound boneless, skinless poultry breasts
1/4 teaspoon black pepper

3 tablespoons balsamic vinegar
3 tablespoons honey
2 teaspoons dried basil
Directions:
Heat olive oil in a skillet over medium heat. Add chook and sprinkle with pepper.
Sauté chook for 5 minutes on each side, until golden brown.
Add balsamic vinegar and sauté for one minute, turning the chook to coat.
Add honey and basil. Stir and turn hen to coat. Cook for one more minute.
Remove to a plate and pour the sauce from the pan over the chook.

Nutritional value:
- Energy value: 153 Kcal
- Protein: 7 g
- Carbohydrates: 16 g
- Fiber: 7 g
- Sugar: 5 g
- Sodium: 2 g
- Fat: 13 g
- Of which:
- - Saturated: 4 g
- - Monounsaturated: 6 g
- - Polyunsaturated: 2 g
- - Cholesterol: 115 mg

143. LEMON AND GARLIC CHICKEN WITH QUINOA AND ORZO

Servings: 4
Ingredients:
2 oz orzo pasta, raw.
2 oz quinoa, uncooked
2 cloves garlic
Half cup onion
1 cup purple bell pepper
1/2 cup fresh mushrooms
12 ounces boneless, skinless poultry breast
2 lemons
1/2 tablespoon loose herb seasoning mix with salt
2 tablespoon halves of olive oil.
Directions:
Cook orzo and quinoa according to package guidelines and reserve.
Mince garlic; chop onion and bell pepper; slice mushrooms.
Cut the chicken into 1" portions. Place chook in a zip-top plastic bag with the juice of 1 lemon and 1 tablespoon of the unsalted herb seasoning blend. Mix all Ingredients: inside the refrigerator.
Heat 1/2 tablespoon olive oil in a medium nonstick skillet over medium heat. Add garlic and onion. Sauté until onion is translucent (three to five minutes). Add bell pepper and mushrooms. Cook, stirring occasionally until peppers are soft (five to seven minutes). Remove from heat and place over low heat.
Heat 1 tablespoon olive oil in a massive nonstick skillet over medium heat. Add the bird and cook dinner till now not pink inside (about 7 minutes).
Mix the final tablespoon of olive oil, the juice of 1 lemon and 1/2 tablespoon of the unsalted herb seasoning mix and load to the hen.
Add the cooked orzo, quinoa and sautéed vegetables, then cook every 3 to five minutes until the chicken is cooked through and all the elements are hot.
Divide slightly to make four servings.

Nutritional value:
- Energy value: 312 Kcal
- Protein: 24 g
- Carbohydrates: 27 g

- Fiber: 3 g
- Sugar: 6g
- Sodium: 46 mg
- Fat: 12 g
- Of which:
- - Saturated: 6g
- - Monounsaturated: 4 g
- - Polyunsaturated: 2 g
- - Cholesterol: 62mg

144. CHICKEN IN SKILLET WITH GREEN BEANS AND POTATOES

Servings: 4
Ingredients:
2 cups of purple potatoes
1 teaspoon olive oil
16 oz. Poultry strips, raw
10 oz. frozen reduced beans, raw
4 tablespoons unsalted butter
1 Tbsp. dry Italian seasoning mix
Directions:
Preheat oven to 4°C. Chop potatoes into small pieces. See helpful hints for potassium discount commands if desired. Toss potatoes in 1 teaspoon olive oil.
Spray a nine x 13-inch baking dish with oil spray. Place raw chicken strips in 1/3 of the pan. Place the potatoes in 1/3 of the pan. Finally, place inexperienced frozen beans in the last 1/3 of the skillet.
Melt the butter and drizzle over the entire skillet of chicken, potatoes and inexperienced beans. Sprinkle the dry Italian dressing mixture over the entire skillet.
Bake for 20 to 30 minutes. Check for doneness after 20 minutes.

Nutritional value:
- Energy value: 137 Kcal
- Protein: 12 g
- Carbohydrates: 13 g
- Fiber: 5 g
- Sugar: 2 g
- Sodium: 2 g
- Fat: 10 g
- Of which:
- - Saturated: 5 g
- - Monounsaturated: 3 g
- - Polyunsaturated: 1 g
- Cholesterol: 153 mg

145. ROAST CHICKEN

Servings: 2
Ingredients:
2 teaspoons olive oil
Whole 3 lb. chicken
1/2 teaspoon kosher salt
1/4 teaspoon black pepper
2 whole garlic heads, cleaned
2 sprigs of rosemary, cleaned
1 lime
Directions:
Preheat oven to 375°F.
Add olive oil to the skillet and begin to heat.
Rinse the inside and outside of the chicken and pat dry.
Sprinkle chicken with salt and pepper, inside and out.
Place 1 whole head of garlic and 2 sprigs of chicken inside the rosemary.

Add chicken to pan and brown on all sides.
After browning, squeeze lime juice over the bird and the exposed area of the pan with the chicken in the oven.
During cooking, periodically pour the juices over the poultry.
Check after 1 hour and half an hour. To see if it is cooked, prick the chicken in the thickest part of the thigh; the juices should run clear.

Nutritional value:
- Energy value: 192 Kcal
- Protein: 19 g
- Carbohydrates: 15 g
- Fiber: 7 g
- Sugar: 3 g
- Sodium: 3 g
- Fat: 10 g
- Of which:
- - Saturated: 5 g
- - Monounsaturated: 3 g
- - Polyunsaturated: 1 g
- - Cholesterol: 127 mg

146. VEGETABLES AND ROASTED ROSEMARY CHICKEN

Servings: 2
Ingredients:
2 medium zucchini
1 medium carrot
1/2 bell pepper
1/2 huge red onion
8 cloves of garlic
1 tablespoon of olive oil
1/4 teaspoon ground pepper
4 bone-in chicken breasts
1 tablespoon dried rosemary
Directions:
Preheat oven to 375°F.
Cut zucchini into 1/2"-thick slices; cut carrot and bell pepper into 1/4"-thick slices; slice onion into 1/2-inch wedges; weigh garlic cloves.
Combine zucchini, carrot, bell pepper, onion, garlic and oil in a thirteen "x nine" roasting pan. Season mixture with 1/2 teaspoon black pepper and toss to coat. Roast until vegetables are heated through, about 10 minutes.
While the vegetables are roasting, lift the pores and skin off the breasts and rub the flesh with black pepper and crumbled rosemary. Replace the skin, after which season the bird with additional pepper and rosemary, as preferred.
Remove the roasting pan from the oven, and near the chicken, pores and skin facets up, at the pinnacle of the vegetables. Return to the oven and continue roasting until the chook is cooked through and the vegetables are tender (approximately 35 minutes).

Nutritional value:
- Energy value: 227 Kcal
- Protein: 5 g
- Carbohydrates: 7 g
- Fiber: 5 g
- Sugar: 3 g
- Sodium: 2 g
- Fat: 9 g
- Of which:
- - Saturated: 7 g
- - Monounsaturated: 1 g
- - Polyunsaturated: 1 g
- - Cholesterol: 100 mg

147. CHICKEN THIGHS IN CLAY POT GLAZE WITH PINEAPPLE

Servings: 5
Ingredients:
1-1 / 2 kilos of boneless and skinless hen thighs.
1/2 teaspoon black pepper
1/2 teaspoon garlic powder
2 tablespoons olive oil
20 small pieces of canned pineapple in unsweetened pineapple juice
2 tablespoons packed brown sugar
2 tablespoons low-sodium soy sauce
Half teaspoon Tabasco® sauce
2 tablespoons cornstarch
3 tablespoons water
4 tablespoons green onions
3 cups cooked rice
Directions:
Sprinkle both sides of the chicken thighs with pepper and garlic powder.
Heat oil in a large skillet over medium-high heat. Add chicken to skillet and cook 2-3 minutes on each facet, until golden brown.
Transfer poultry to a four-quart casserole dish coated with cooking spray.
Drain pineapple juice into a measuring cup. If you have less than 1 cup, add water to make 1 cup. Stir the juice into the fat in the pan and scrape to loosen the browned chicken pieces. Remove from heat and stir in brown sugar, soy sauce and Tabasco sauce. Add 1 cup pineapple chunks. Pour the aggregate over the poultry thighs in a crockpot. Cover and simmer on low heat for three hours.
Remove poultry from crockpot and turn heat to high. Combine cornstarch and three tablespoons of water in a small bowl. Add the sauce into the crockpot. Cook for 2 minutes or until sauce thickens, stirring continuously with a whisk. Add green onions and stir to coat. Serve each chicken thigh over 1/2 cup of rice.

Nutritional value:
- Energy value: 175 Kcal
- Protein: 13 g
- Carbohydrates: 11 g
- Fiber: 3 g
- Sugar: 2 g
- Sodium: 3 g
- Fat: 11 g
- Of which:
- - Saturated: 3 g
- - Monounsaturated: 5 g
- - Polyunsaturated: 2 g
- - Cholesterol: 87 mg

148. ROASTED CHICKEN, ASPARAGUS AND CORN

Servings: 4
Ingredients:
8 oz. boneless, skinless chicken breast (1 large breast or 2 medium breasts)
2 tablespoons olive oil
1/2 teaspoon ground black pepper
1/2 teaspoon mixed herbs and spices (cumin, paprika, chili powder)
1/4 teaspoon crushed purple pepper flakes
10 asparagus spears
1 ear of fresh corn on the cob (Colorado corn if available)
1/2 lime
1 tablespoon sparkling chives
Starting

Season the poultry breast with 1 tablespoon olive oil, ground black pepper, mixed herbs and spices and crushed pink pepper flakes. Add the hen to the hot spot on the grill, side down. Grill for 12 minutes. While the chicken is cooking, slice the asparagus and place it on the grill. Season with black pepper and drizzle with 2 teaspoons olive oil. Grill the asparagus for five to 7 minutes.
Cut corn on the cob in half and drizzle with 1 teaspoon olive oil. Grill the corn for three to four minutes, until lightly charred. After removing the corn from the grill, add a squeeze of lemon juice and chopped scallions.
Squeeze the lemon over the chicken and asparagus to taste.

Nutritional value:
- Energy value: 338 Kcal
- Protein: 30g
- Carbohydrates: 14 g
- Fiber: 4 g
- Sugar: 5 g
- Sodium: 58 mg
- Fat: 18g
- Of which:
- - Saturated: 8g
- - Monounsaturated: 5 g
- - Polyunsaturated: 5 g
- - Cholesterol: 83 mg

149. FETA PASTA WITH CHICKEN AND ASPARAGUS

Servings: 5
Ingredients:
1 pound thin asparagus spears
8 ounces boneless, skinless chicken breasts
16 ounces penne pasta, uncooked
5 tablespoons olive oil
1/4 teaspoon black pepper
1/4 teaspoon garlic powder
1/2 cup low-sodium chicken broth
1 clove garlic
1-1 / 2 teaspoons dried oregano
1/4 cup crumbled feta cheese
Directions:
Trim asparagus and cut diagonally into 1 " pieces. Cut the ken chic into cubes.
Bring a large pot of water to a boil. Add the pasta and cook as directed on the box or about 8 to 10 minutes. Do not add salt. Drain and set aside.
Heat 3 tablespoons olive oil in a large skillet over medium-high heat. Add chicken and season with pepper and garlic powder. Cook until chicken is cooked through and browned, about 5 minutes. Remove chicken to paper towels.
Pour the chicken broth into the skillet. Add the asparagus, minced garlic, a pinch more garlic powder, oregano and pepper.
Cover and steam until asparagus are tender, about 5 minutes.
Return the chicken to the skillet and heat through.
Add chicken mixture to pasta and mix well. Let stand for about 5 minutes.
Drizzle with remaining 2 tablespoons olive oil, toss again and then sprinkle with feta cheese.

Nutritional value:
- Energy value: 192 Kcal
- Protein: 19 g
- Carbohydrates: 15 g
- Fiber: 7 g
- Sugar: 3 g
- Sodium: 3 g
- Fat: 10 g
- Of which:
- - Saturated: 5 g

- •   - Monounsaturated: 3 g
- •   - Polyunsaturated: 1 g
-   - Cholesterol: 127 mg

150. RICE AND CHICKEN STEW LOUISIANA STYLE

Servings: 5
Ingredients:
3 cups of cooked white rice
6 chicken wings
6 chicken thighs
1/2 cup onion
3/4 cup green bell pepper
3 cloves garlic
2 tablespoons vegetable oil
2 tablespoons all-purpose flour
1/4 teaspoon black pepper
1 pinch pink pepper
Half cup low sodium chook broth
Half cup water
Directions:
Prepare rice according to Directions: on package omitting salt.
Chop onion and bell peppers; mince garlic.
Rinse chook parts with bloodless water. Pat dry with paper towels.
Heat oil in a skillet or saucepan; Bring up browned chook chicken parts all over.
Add onion and green bell pepper.
Sprinkle flour over vegetables and hen items, stirring to coat all pieces.
Let the hen and flour brown for about five minutes.
Stir in garlic, black pepper and pink pepper.
Add broth and water.
Cover the pot and simmer for about 30 minutes or until the chicken is cooked through. (The sauce will thicken as it simmers).
Serve over white rice.

Nutritional Value	
• Energy value: 245 Kcal	
• Protein: 25g	
• Carbohydrates: 21 g	
• Fiber: 2 g	
• Sugar: 2g	
• Sodium: 1g	
• Fat: 6g	
• Of which:	
• - Saturated: 2 g	
• - Monounsaturated: 2 g	
• - Polyunsaturated: 2g	
• - Cholesterol: 35 mg	

151. TURKEY MEATLOAF

Servings: 5
Ingredients:
1 pound of ground turkey, 7% fat
3 oz. Turkey sausage
1 whole egg
1 egg white
1/2 cup dry bread crumbs
1/4 cup clean parsley, chopped
1 tablespoon Worcestershire sauce
1 teaspoon Gravy Master browning and seasoning sauce
1 teaspoon Italian seasoning
1/2 teaspoon black pepper
Directions:

Preheat oven to 350°F.
Combine all substances in a large bowl and mix well.
Transfer to a greased 9 "x 5" loaf pan and bake for 1 hour.
Cut into 6 equal portions and serve.

Nutritional value:	
• Energy value: 192 Kcal	
• Protein: 19 g	
• Carbohydrates: 15 g	
• Fiber: 7 g	
• Sugar: 3 g	
• Sodium: 3 g	
• Fat: 10 g	
• Of which:	
• - Saturated: 5 g	
• - Monounsaturated: 3 g	
• - Polyunsaturated: 1 g	
• - Cholesterol: 127 mg	

152. EASY RIBS

Servings: 5
Ingredients:
Garlic-Herb Seasoning, 1 teaspoon Mix together.
Pork ribs, 1 1/2 pounds
3 quarts liquid
1/2 gallon of apple cider vinegar
1/4 cup barbecue sauce
Directions:
seasoning should be evenly distributed on both the top and bottom of the ribs.
Coat the top of a roasting pan with cooking spray and place the ribs on top.
Fill the bottom of the roasting pan with water and vinegar. Place the ribs on top of the pan.
Cover the ribs with aluminum foil, tucking in the edges. (You may need two pieces of foil to cover everything). The ribs will steam as a result.
Bake for 3-1/2 to 4 hours at 300°F; do not watch because it will release steam.
Brush with barbecue sauce after removing foil. Cook for another 10 minutes in the oven.

Nutritional value	
• Energy value:282 Kcal	
• Protein: 34g	
• Carbohydrates: 6 g	
• Fiber: 1g	
• Sugar: 2g	
• Sodium: 381 mg	
• Fat: 13g	
• Of which:	
• - Saturated: 7 g	
• - Monounsaturated: 3 g	
• - Polyunsaturated: 3g	
Cholesterol: 100 mg	

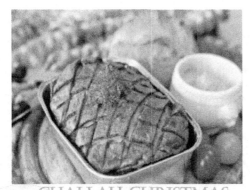

153.   CHALLAH CHRISTMAS DRESS

Servings: 5
Ingredients:
2 pounds of Jala bread
2 medium onions
4 celery stalks
2 medium green peppers
2 medium carrots
4 cloves garlic
5 tablespoons unsalted butter
2 tablespoons poultry seasoning
1 pound ground turkey, 7% fat
2 cups low sodium turkey broth
3 large eggs
1/2 cup fresh parsley
Directions:
Cut the challah loaves into pieces and let them rest overnight.
Preheat oven to 350°F. Chop onion, celery, green peppers, carrots and parsley. Mince the garlic.
In a large skillet, heat 4 tablespoons butter until lightly browned.
Add ground turkey and sauté until browned. Remove turkey from skillet and set aside to cool.
Add onion, celery, green peppers and carrots to the same skillet and sauté until tender. Add garlic and heat for 1 to 2 minutes more.
Grease an oven-safe skillet with the remaining tablespoon of butter. Sprinkle the poultry seasoning over the bread pieces and add to the skillet.
Beat the eggs and mix with the cooled turkey mixture.
Add the egg-turkey mixture and 1/4 cup chopped parsley to the bread. Mix gently.
Add turkey broth and stir to combine. The mixture will be mushy.
Cover the pan and bake for 40 minutes. Remove the lid and bake for 20 minutes more.
Sprinkle remaining parsley on top before serving.

Nutritional value:
• Energy value: 175 Kcal
• Protein: 13 g
• Carbohydrates: 11 g
• Fiber: 3 g
• Sugar: 2 g
• Sodium: 3 g
• Fat: 11 g
• Of which:
• - Saturated: 3 g
• - Monounsaturated: 5 g
• - Polyunsaturated: 2 g
- Cholesterol: 87 mg

154.   EGGPLANT WITH MEATBALLS (BORANI BADEMJAN)

Servings: 5
Ingredients:
1 clove garlic
Yellow bell pepper, 1/2 cup
2 eggplants (medium)
1 pound of onion
A fraction of a cup of canola oil
1 pound of ground beef, lean
1 tablespoon of turmeric powder
1 teaspoon lemon pepper (unsalted)
1 tablespoon Mrs. Dash® seasoning mix
1 cup tomato sauce
2 cups of water
Directions:
Garlic cloves should be peeled and crushed. The green bell pepper should be thinly sliced and the onion should be finely diced. Peel the eggplant and cut it lengthwise before cutting it into pieces.
Heat the oil in a non-stick frying pan and add the crushed garlic and green bell pepper. Remove the item and set it aside.
Sauté the eggplant on both sides in the same oil until golden brown. Remove and set aside.
Combine ground beef, onion and spices in a mixing bowl. Create a total of 30 small meatballs.
In a non-stick skillet, brown the meatballs over low heat (do not use oil).
Toss meatballs with sautéed eggplant, garlic, bell pepper, crushed stewed tomatoes and water. Simmer for 30 minutes at low pressure.

Nutritional value:
• Energy value: 153 Kcal
• Protein: 7 g
• Carbohydrates: 16 g
• Fiber: 7 g
• Sugar: 5 g
• Sodium: 2 g
• Fat: 13 g
• Of which:
• - Saturated: 4 g
• - Monounsaturated: 6 g
• - Polyunsaturated: 2 g
• - Cholesterol: 115 mg

155.   GROUND BEEF AND VEGETABLE DINNER IN FOIL PACKET

Servings: 5
Ingredients:
4 ounces of beef (ground)
1 tablespoon onion
Worcestershire sauce, 1 tablespoon
3/4 cup carrots and peas, frozen
1 tablespoon dry Italian dressing mix
1 teaspoon cayenne pepper.
Directions:
Preheat oven to 375°F. With nonstick cooking spray, coat a piece of aluminum foil. Finely chop the onion.
Form a patty with the ground beef, onion and Worcestershire sauce and place on the foil.
The frozen peas and carrots go on top of the patty.
In the end, sprinkle with the Italian dressing mixture and black pepper.

Place foil on a baking sheet after folding and sealing. Preheat oven to 350°F and bake for 35 minutes.

Until ready to serve, carefully open one end of the foil packet and allow steam to escape.

Nutritional value:
- Energy value: 192 Kcal
- Protein: 19 g
- Carbohydrates: 15 g
- Fiber: 7 g
- Sugar: 3 g
- Sodium: 3 g
- Fat: 10 g
- Of which:
- - Saturated: 5 g
- - Monounsaturated: 3 g
- - Polyunsaturated: 1 g
- Cholesterol: 127 mg

156. GRILLED SKIRT STEAK AND VEGETABLES WITH VINAIGRETTE

Servings: 5
Ingredients:
Flank steak, 1 lb.
Half teaspoon salt
1 teaspoon freshly ground black pepper
1 medium eggplant
2 bell peppers, medium
6 tablespoons extra virgin olive oil, extra virgin
2 tablespoons balsamic vinaigrette
1 clove garlic
1/4 cup flat-leaf parsley, new

Directions:
Preheat grill to medium-high heat.
You can use 1/4 teaspoon salt and 1/2 teaspoon pepper to season the steak.
Grill until done to your liking, about 4 to 5 minutes per side for medium-rare.
Until sliced, transfer to a cutting board and let rest for at least 5 minutes.
While the steak is cooking, quarter and seed the bell peppers and slice the eggplant into four 1/2"-thick rounds.
3 tablespoons oil, rubbed on both sides of the eggplant and peppers
1/4 teaspoon salt and 1/2 teaspoon pepper to taste.
4 to 5 minutes per side on the grill until tender.
The garlic cloves should be minced and the parsley should be chopped. To make a vinaigrette sauce, mix the remaining oil, vinegar, garlic and parsley in a small bowl.
In 4 shallow dishes, divide the steak and vegetables.
Serve the sauce on the side or over the vegetables.

Nutritional value:
- Energy value: 345 kcal
- Protein: 28 g
- Carbohydrates: 8 g
- Fiber: 2 g
- Sugar: 5 g
- Sodium: 533 mg
- Fat: 22 g
- Of which:
- - Saturated: 6 g
- - Monounsaturated: 13 g
- - Polyunsaturated: 3 g
- - Cholesterol: 76 mg

157. HOMEMADE SAUSAGE IN PAN

Servings: 5
Ingredients:
1 pound ground red meat
2 teaspoons ground sage
2 teaspoons sugar or sugar substitute
1 teaspoon basil, dried and crushed
1-1 / 2 teaspoons black pepper
1/4 teaspoon ground red bell pepper.

Directions:
In an enormous bowl, mix all elements collectively.
Divide into 8 identical portions and shape into individual empanadas.
Cook or freeze for later use.

Nutritional value:
- Energy value: 153 Kcal
- Protein: 7 g
- Carbohydrates: 16 g
- Fiber: 7 g
- Sugar: 5 g
- Sodium: 2 g
- Fat: 13 g
- Of which:
- - Saturated: 4 g
- - Monounsaturated: 6 g
- - Polyunsaturated: 2 g - Cholesterol: 115 mg

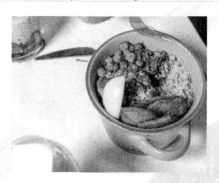

158. QUICK AND EASY CHICKEN SAUTÉ

Servings: 5
Ingredients:
8 ounces of cooked poultry breast
3 tablespoons canola oil
10-ounce bag broccoli slaw
1/3 cup hoisin sauce
1/3 cup water

Directions:
Shred-cooked chicken breast.
In a large wok, heat 1 tablespoon oil and whisk in broccoli slaw; prepare dinner for 5 minutes.
Add hoisin sauce, water and final 2 tablespoons oil to wok. Stir collectively.
Add shredded chook to wok. Toss chicken and broccoli salad.
Serve over rice or rice noodles if desired.

Nutritional value:
- Energy value: 192 Kcal
- Protein: 19 g
- Carbohydrates: 15 g
- Fiber: 7 g
- Sugar: 3 g
- Sodium: 3 g
- Fat: 10 g

- Of which:
  - - Saturated: 5 g
  - - Monounsaturated: 3 g
  - - Polyunsaturated: 1 g
- - Cholesterol: 127 mg

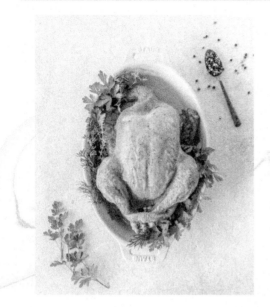

159.   CHICKEN DINNER WITH LEMON AND CILANTRO

Servings: 2
Ingredients:
1 cup uncooked jasmine rice
3/4 cup cilantro
1/2 cup lime juice
2 tablespoons fresh ginger
1 half teaspoon lime peel
Half teaspoon pepper
Half teaspoon salt
1 pound boneless, skinless breasts
2 tablespoons canola oil
3 small zucchini

Directions:
Prepare the rice according to orders but pass the salt. Chop cilantro; chop ginger and lime zest.
In a small bowl, stir together cilantro, ginger, lime zest, 1/4 teaspoon pepper, salt and lime juice. Place breasts in a zip-lock bag and pour in half of the marinade. Marinate the chicken in the refrigerator for 30 to 60 minutes. Place the best cilantro mixture in a screw-top pinnacle jar and set it aside as a dressing.
Heat a solid iron skillet with large rims over medium heat. Drizzle chicken with 2 teaspoons of oil. Place in hot skillet and cook four to five minutes per facet or until cooked through.
While the chicken is cooking, cut the zucchini into quarters, lengthwise and toss with the final pepper and oil. Cook in a grill pan, turning frequently, for 10 minutes or until golden brown and crisp-tender. Cover with foil until ready to serve.

Divide rice among 4 bowls. Cut poultry into thick strips and place on top of rice. Shake dressing well and drizzle over chicken. Serve with zucchini.

Nutritional value:
- Energy value: 272 Kcal
- Protein: 36 g
- Carbohydrates: 13 g
- Fiber: 1 g
- Sugar: 1 g
- Sodium: 106 mg
- Fat: 7 g
- Of which:
- - Saturated: 2 g
- - Monounsaturated: 3 g
- - Polyunsaturated: 2 g
- - Cholesterol: 82 mg

160.   ROASTED TURKEY BREAST WITH SALT-FREE HERB SEASONING

Servings: 5
Ingredients:
3 pounds fresh turkey breast 1/2, bone in, with pores and skin.
1/4 cup butter
1 tablespoon salt-free herb seasoning blend
1/4 cup onion

Directions:
Preheat oven to 350° F.
Finely chop the onion. Melt butter, then add onion and herb seasoning combination. Divide the mixture in 1/2.
In a large roasting pan or skillet, place the turkey breast pores, skin side down. Top with 1 tablespoon of the seasoning rub.
Turn the breast over and loosen pores and skin with palms. Spread 3 tablespoons of the seasoning blend between the meat and skin. Use toothpicks to connect the edges of the skin to the breast meat.
Place the skillet inside the oven and bake for 1 hour.
Remove the skillet from the oven and spread the final seasoning mixture over the turkey skin.
Return the skillet to the oven and prepare dinner for 15 to twenty minutes or until the meat thermometer reads 160° F.
Remove the skillet from the oven and let the turkey breast rest for 10-15 minutes before carving.

Nutritional value:
- Energy value: 203 Kcal
- Protein: 25g
- Carbohydrates: 1 g
- Fiber: 0g
- Sugar: 0 g
- Sodium:88 m g
- Fat: 4 g
- Of which:
- - Saturated:2 g
- - Monounsaturated: 1 g
- - Polyunsaturated: 1 g
- - Cholesterol: 76 mg

DESSERTS:

161. PROTEIN-BOOSTING BLUEBERRY MUFFINS

Servings: 5
Ingredients:
1 cup oat flakes
1 cup plain non-fat Greek yogurt
Half cup olive oil
1/4 cup water
3/4 cup brown sugar
1 large egg
1 cup all-purpose flour
1-1 / three cups of whey protein powder
1/2 teaspoon salt
1/2 teaspoon baking soda
1/2 teaspoon of cream of tartar
1 cup cleaned blueberries
Directions:
Preheat oven to 350°F.
In a large bowl, mix oats with yogurt. Add oil, water, sugar and egg; mix well.
In a separate bowl, integrate flour, protein powder, salt, baking soda and cream of tartar.
Mix Ingredients: dry into wet ingredients. Add blueberries and mix well.
Fill 12 muffin pans or grease muffin pans and fill 2/3 full with batter.
Bake for 20 to 25 minutes or until firm to the touch.

Nutritional value:
- Energy value: 175 Kcal
- Protein: 13 g
- Carbohydrates: 11 g
- Fiber: 3 g
- Sugar: 2 g
- Sodium: 3 g
- Fat: 11 g
- Of which:
- - Saturated: 3 g
- - Monounsaturated: 5 g
- - Polyunsaturated: 2 g
- - Cholesterol: 87 mg

162. JACKIE'S CORNBREAD MUFFINS

Servings: 2
Ingredients:
1 cup white all-purpose flour
1 cup undeniable corn flour, white or yellow
1/4 cup sugar
2 teaspoons baking powder
1/2 cup liquid egg replacement
1 cup rice milk, un-enriched
2 tablespoons unsalted butter, melted, or 2 tablespoons canola oil
Directions:
Preheat oven to four hundred ° F.
In a bowl, integrate the flour, cornmeal, sugar and baking powder.
In any other bowl, combine the egg substitute, rice milk and melted butter.
Stir the dry substances into the wet items until moistened.
Fill greased or paper-lined muffin tins 2/3 full.

Bake 15 to 20 minutes or until a toothpick comes out clean. Serve warm.

Nutritional value:
- Energy value: 153 Kcal
- Protein: 7 g
- Carbohydrates: 16 g
- Fiber: 7 g
- Sugar: 5 g
- Sodium: 2 g
- Fat: 13 g
- Of which:
- - Saturated: 4 g
- - Monounsaturated: 6 g
- - Polyunsaturated: 2 g
- - Cholesterol: 115 mg

163. EGG MUFFINS

Servings: 5
Ingredients:
1 cup bell peppers (red, yellow and orange).
1 cup of onion
Half pound of red meat
1/4 teaspoon of rooster seasoning
1/4 teaspoon garlic powder
1/4 teaspoon of onion powder
1/2 teaspoon Mrs. Dash® herb seasoning mix
8 large eggs
2 tablespoons milk or milk substitute
1/4 teaspoon salt (optional)
Directions:
Preheat oven to 350°F and spray an everyday size muffin pan with cooking spray.
Finely chop bell peppers and onion.
In a bowl, combine the red meat, rooster seasoning, garlic powder, onion powder and Mrs. Dash seasoning to make the sausage.
In a nonstick skillet, prepare sausage for dinner until done; drain.
Beat eggs together with milk or milk substitute and salt.
Add sausage crumbs and vegetables; mix.
Pour egg aggregate into organized muffin tins, leaving room for truffles to push up. Bake for 18 to 22 minutes.

Nutritional value:
- Energy value: 139 Kcal
- Protein: 11g
- Carbohydrates: 2 g
- Fiber: 1g
- Sugar: 1g
- Sodium: 182 mg
- Fat: 10 g
- Of which:
- - Saturated: 5 g
- - Monounsaturated: 2 g
- - Polyunsaturated: 3g
- - Cholesterol: 245 mg

164. PUFFED BAKED PANCAKE

Servings: 1
Ingredients:
2 tablespoons butter
2 large eggs
Half cup rice flour
Half cup rice milk
1/8 teaspoon salt
Directions:
Preheat oven to 400°F.
Place butter in a 10-inch ovenproof skillet or glass pie plate. Place in oven for three to 5 minutes or until butter is melted.
In a medium mixing bowl, use a wire whisk or rotary beater to beat the eggs until combined. Add the rice flour, rice milk and salt. Whisk until smooth.
Remove the pan or cake pan from the oven. Immediately pour the batter into the new pan. Bake for 25 to 30 minutes until the pancake is puffed and nicely browned.
Transfer to a serving dish and reduce to 4 quantities. Add toppings of choice. Serve hot.

Nutritional value:
- Energy value: 131Kcal
- Protein: 5 g
- Carbohydrates:12 g
- Fiber: 1g
- Sugar: 4g
- Sodium: 41mg
- Fat: 6g
- Of which:
- - Saturated: 3 g
- - Monounsaturated: 2 g
- - Polyunsaturated: 1g
- - Cholesterol: 117 mg

165. FRESH FRUIT DESSERT CUPS

Servings: 5
Ingredients:
4 sheets of puff pastry dough, 14" x 18."
Non-stick cooking spray, butter flavored
1 cup sparkling blueberries
1 cup fresh blackberries
1 cup cleaned raspberries
1 cup fresh strawberries
3 cups Cool Whip frozen dessert topping
Directions:
Preheat oven to 400°F.
Spray a 12-cup muffin tin with Pam butter-flavored cooking spray.
Place 4 sheets of phyllo dough together, spraying lightly with cooking spray between each layer. Cut the phyllo dough into three halves of squares and area in a muffin tin to make dessert cups.
Place the muffin pan in the oven and bake for 10 to 12 minutes or until the phyllo cups are lightly browned. Let cool to room temperature.
When ready to serve, fill each phyllo dessert cup with 1/3 cup of sparkling berries. Top with 1/4 cup Cool Whip dessert topping.

Nutritional value:
- Energy value: 192 Kcal
- Protein: 19 g
- Carbohydrates: 15 g
- Fiber: 7 g
- Sugar: 3 g
- Sodium: 3 g
- Fat: 10 g

- Of which:
- - Saturated: 5 g
- - Monounsaturated: 3 g
- - Polyunsaturated: 1 g
- - Cholesterol: 127 mg

166. QUICK AND EASY APPLE AND OATMEAL CUSTARD

Servings: 1
Ingredients:
1/2 medium apple
1/3 cup quick-cooking oatmeal
1 large egg, whisked
1/2 cup almond milk
1/4 teaspoon cinnamon
Directions:
Core and finely chop half of an apple.
Combine oatmeal and almond milk in a large bowl. Stir well with a fork. Add the cinnamon and apple. Stir once more until completely blended.
Microwave at excessive heat for 2 minutes.
Stir with a fork. Cook 30 to 60 seconds longer if necessary.
Add the whisked egg to the mixture and stir until well combined
Add a little water if a thinner cereal is desired.

Nutritional value:
- Energy value: 152 Kcal
- Protein: 9 g
- Carbohydrates: 15 g
- Fiber: 7 g
- Sugar: 3 g
- Sodium: 3 g
- Fat: 10 g
- Of which:
- - Saturated: 5 g
- - Monounsaturated: 3 g
- - Polyunsaturated: 1 g
- - Cholesterol: 121 mg

167. EASY LOW PHOSPHORUS FUDGE

Servings: 1
Ingredients:
2/3 cup, half and 1/2 cream
1-2/3 cups granulated sugar
1-1 / 2 cups miniature marshmallows
1/2 cup semisweet chocolate chips
1 teaspoon vanilla extract
Directions:
Grease a 9" rectangular pan with nonstick spray or butter.
Combine half-and-half and half of the sugar in a large heavy saucepan. Bring to a boil; reduce heat to medium. Stir constantly and continue to boil for 5 minutes.
Remove pan from heat and load in marshmallows, chocolate chips and vanilla extract. Stir until marshmallows are melted.
Quickly pour into greased pan. Cool; cut into three "x 1 half" pieces, making 18 servings.

Nutritional value:
- Energy value: 153 Kcal
- Protein: 7 g
- Carbohydrates: 16 g
- Fiber: 7 g
- Sugar: 5 g
- Sodium: 2 g
- Fat: 13 g
- Of which:

- Saturated: 4 g
- Monounsaturated: 6 g
- Polyunsaturated: 2 g
- Cholesterol: 115 mg

168. EASY APPLE AND OAT CRISP

Servings: 5
Ingredients:
5 Granny Smith apples
1 cup whole oats
3/4 cup brown sugar
1/2 cup all-purpose flour
1 teaspoon cinnamon
1/2 cup butter
Directions:
Preheat oven to 350°F. Peel, core and slice apples.
In a bowl, mix oats, brown sugar, flour and cinnamon.

Cut the butter into the oat combination with a pastry cutter until well blended.
Place sliced apples in a nine "x 9" baking pan.
Sprinkle the oat mixture over the apples.
Bake for 30 to 35 minutes.

Nutritional value:
- Energy value:110 Kcal
- Protein: 1 g
- Carbohydrates: 17 g
- Fiber: 1g
- Sugar: 0g
- Sodium: 85 mg
- Fat: 5g
- Of which:
- - Saturated: 2 g
- - Monounsaturated: 2 g
- - Polyunsaturated: 1 g
- - Cholesterol: 11 mg

Bases:

169. PUMPKIN AND CRANBERRY BREAD

Servings: 5
Ingredients:
1 cup oat flakes
1 cup plain non-fat Greek yogurt
Half cup olive oil
1/4 cup water
3/4 cup brown sugar
1 large egg
1 cup plain flour
1-1/3 cups whey protein powder
1/2 teaspoon salt
1/2 teaspoon baking soda
1/2 teaspoon of cream of tartar
1 cup cleaned blueberries

Directions:
Preheat oven to 350°F.
In a large bowl, mix oats with yogurt. Add oil, water, sugar and egg; mix well.
In a separate bowl, combine flour, protein powder, salt, baking soda and cream of tartar.
Mix dry ingredients into wet ingredients. Add blueberries and mix well.
Fill 12 muffin pans or grease muffin pans and fill 2/3 full with batter.
Bake for 20 to 25 minutes or until firm to the touch.

Nutritional value:
- Energy value: 153Kcal
- Protein: 3g
- Carbohydrates: 35 g
- Fiber: 1g
- Sugar: 22g
- Sodium: 272 mg
- Fat: 0g
- Of which:
- - Saturated: 0 g
- - Monounsaturated: 0 g
- - Polyunsaturated: 0g
- - Cholesterol: 0mg

170. APPLE AND ZUCCHINI BREAD

Servings: 5
Ingredients:
3-three / four cups plus 2 tablespoons flour for all motifs.
1 cup Granny Smith apples
2 cups zucchini
4 huge eggs
1/2 cup vegetable oil
3/4 cup granulated sugar
1 cup brown sugar
1 teaspoon vanilla extract
1-1/2 teaspoons baking soda
1/2 teaspoon salt
Three teaspoons cinnamon on the ground
2 tablespoons cold unsalted butter
Directions:

Preheat oven to 350° F. Grease and flour two 9 "x 5" loaf pans with 2 tablespoons flour.
Peel and chop apples; grate zucchini.
In a large bowl, mix eggs, oil, granulated sugar, 3/4 cup brown sugar (or 6 tablespoons Splenda brown sugar mixture) and vanilla.
In a separate large bowl, mix together baking soda, 3 1/2 cups flour, salt and a couple of teaspoons cinnamon.
Add the flour mixture to the egg mixture. Now do not over mix.
Fold in the apples and zucchini and pour the aggregate into loaf pans. Spread the mixture calmly.
Bake for forty minutes.
While the bread is baking, prepare the crumb topping: integrate the last 1/4 cup flour, 1/4 cup brown sugar (or 2 tablespoons Splenda brown sugar combination) and 1 teaspoon cinnamon. Cut into the butter until the aggregate becomes very crumbly.
Take the bread from the oven as soon as it has baked for forty minutes and add the crumbs.
Bake for 10 more minutes or until a toothpick (from the center of the loaf) comes out easily.
Let cool for 10 minutes, then remove loaves from pans and transfer to racks to cool completely.
Cut each loaf into eighteen 1/2" slices before serving.

Nutritional value:
- Energy value: 153 Kcal
- Protein: 7 g
- Carbohydrates: 16 g
- Fiber: 7 g
- Sugar: 5 g
- Sodium: 2 g
- Fat: 13 g
- Of which:
- - Saturated: 4 g
- - Monounsaturated: 6 g
- - Polyunsaturated: 2 g
- - Cholesterol: 115 mg

171. LEMON AND BERRY BREAD

Servings: 5
Ingredients:
1-1 / 2 cups white all-purpose flour
1 teaspoon baking powder
1/3 cup canola oil
2/3 cup granulated white sugar
2 tablespoons lemon extract
4 egg whites
1/2 cup 1% fat-free milk
1 cup cleaned blueberries
3/4 cup powdered sugar
1/4 cup lemon juice
1 tablespoon grated lemon zest
Directions:
Preheat oven to 350 ° F. Coat a 9 x 5-inch loaf pan with cooking spray and ground with flour.
In a large bowl, combine flour and baking powder.
In another bowl, mix oil, granulated sugar, milk, lemon extract and egg whites.
Add the flour mixture to the oil and sugar combination. Stir until blended; no longer overmix.
Stir in blueberries and lemon zest.

Pour batter into a loaf pan and bake for 40 to 50 minutes or until a toothpick comes out easily as soon as inserted.

Prepare the glaze while the bread bakes. In a small saucepan, combine the powdered sugar and lemon juice. Heat until the sugar dissolves.

After removing the bread from the oven, without delay poke holes at 1-inch intervals in the pinnacle and pour the lemon glaze over the bread.

Nutritional value:
- Energy value: 175 Kcal
- Protein: 13 g
- Carbohydrates: 11 g
- Fiber: 3 g
- Sugar: 2 g
- Sodium: 3 g
- Fat: 11 g
- Of which:
- - Saturated: 3 g
- - Monounsaturated: 5 g
- - Polyunsaturated: 2 g
- Cholesterol: 87 mg

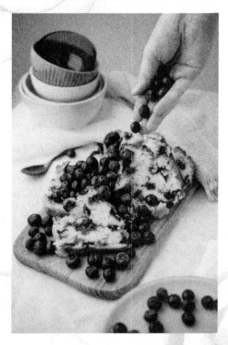

172. LEMON AND PEPPER HUMMUS

Servings: 5
Ingredients:
30 oz of canned chickpeas, canned (2 cans)
1/3 cup extra virgin olive oil
One lemon
1 teaspoon lemon-pepper seasoning (unsalted)
1/8 teaspoon garlic powder
Directions:
Place the chickpeas in a food processor or blender after draining and rinsing.

Reserve 1 tablespoon of olive oil. Combine the chickpeas with the remaining olive oil, lemon juice, lemon pepper seasoning and garlic powder.

Blend or process until smooth. If necessary, thin with 2 to 3 tablespoons of water.

Place in a bowl and drizzle with the remaining tablespoon of olive oil.

Nutritional value:
- Energy value: 192 Kcal

- Protein: 19 g
- Carbohydrates: 15 g
- Fiber: 7 g
- Sugar: 3 g
- Sodium: 3 g
- Fat: 10 g
- Of which:
- - Saturated: 5 g
- - Monounsaturated: 3 g
- - Polyunsaturated: 1 g
- Cholesterol: 127 mg

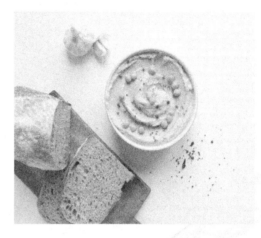

173. PINEAPPLE AND SWEET ONION SALSA WITH TORTILLA CHIPS

Servings: 6
Ingredients:
1/3 cup chopped cilantro
1 medium sweet onion 1/2 small jalapeño bell pepper
2 medium 12 oz canned pineapple crushed in canned juice
1/2 teaspoon lime zest
Ten 6" diameter flour tortillas
4 tablespoons margarine (trans-fat-free)
Directions:
Preheat oven to 375°F.

Remove seeds from jalapeño bell pepper and coarsely chop cilantro and onion.

Combine cilantro, jalapeño and onion in a food processor. Blend until smooth, but not pureed.

Combine the quartered tomatoes with the rest of the ingredients. Pulse until tomatoes break into small pieces.

Pulse the drained pineapple until the mixture is thickened but not pureed.

Add the lemon zest. Blend until well combined.

With melted margarine, brush the four tortillas.

Each tortilla should be cut into 8 pie-shaped pieces. Place on a baking sheet that has been lightly sprayed.

Toasted tortillas should be firm after 10-12 minutes in the oven. Remove from oven and allow to cool.

Baked tortilla pieces can be used as spoonfuls for dipping sauce.

Nutritional value:
- Energy value: 192 Kcal
- Protein: 19 g
- Carbohydrates: 15 g
- Fiber: 7 g
- Sugar: 3 g
- Sodium: 3 g
- Fat: 10 g
- Of which:

- - Saturated: 5 g
- - Monounsaturated: 3 g
- - Polyunsaturated: 1 g
- - Cholesterol: 127 mg

174. CREAM CHEESE DIP WITH MINT JELLY

Servings: 5
Ingredients:
8 ounces cream cheese
1/2 cup mint jelly
30 low sodium crackers
Directions:
Open the cream cheese and place the entire stick on a serving plate.
Spread the jelly on top of the cream cheese.
Serve with low-sodium crackers or flatbread.

Nutritional value:
- Energy value: 227 Kcal
- Protein: 5 g
- Carbohydrates: 7 g
- Fiber: 5 g
- Sugar: 3 g
- Sodium: 2 g
- Fat: 9 g
- Of which:
- - Saturated: 7 g
- - Monounsaturated: 1 g
- - Polyunsaturated: 1 g
- - Cholesterol: 100 mg

175. CHEESE DIP

Servings: 5
Ingredients:
1 1/2 cups cottage cheese (optional)
1 gallon of sour cream
3 onions (green)
2 teaspoons Tabasco chili sauce
1 teaspoon of dill (dill)
1/4 teaspoon garlic powder
1/3 cup blue cheese, crumbled.
Directions:
In a food processor, combine cottage cheese, sour cream, green onions, hot sauce and spices until smooth.
Process for a few seconds after adding the blue cheese.
If necessary, garnish with chopped green onions.

Nutritional value:
- Energy value: 175 Kcal
- Protein: 13 g
- Carbohydrates: 11 g
- Fiber: 3 g
- Sugar: 2 g
- Sodium: 3 g
- Fat: 11 g
- Of which:
- - Saturated: 3 g
- - Monounsaturated: 5 g
- - Polyunsaturated: 2 g
- - Cholesterol: 87 mg

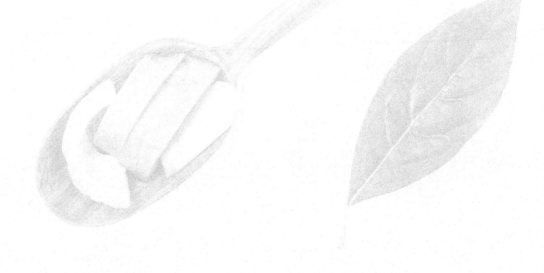

DRINKS:

176. PARTY PUNCH (LOW SUGAR)

Servings: 4
Ingredients:
1/2 cup fruit punch concentrate (liquid)
1 liter of diet lemon-lime soft drink
1 pint of sherbet (lime or lemon)
Directions:
Fill a punch bowl or large mixing bowl half full with soda.
Add fruit punch concentrate.
The sherbet is added with an ice cream scoop.
Add sherbet as it begins to melt and serve.

Nutritional value:
- Energy value: 192 Kcal
- Protein: 19 g
- Carbohydrates: 15 g
- Fiber: 7 g
- Sugar: 3 g
- Sodium: 3 g
- Fat: 10 g
- Of which:
- - Saturated: 5 g
- - Monounsaturated: 3 g
- - Polyunsaturated: 1 g
- - Cholesterol: 127 mg

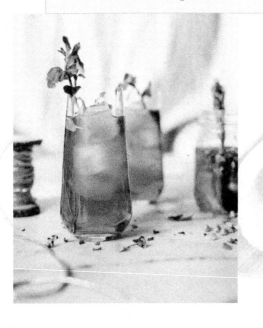

177. HOT WASSAIL (CIDER)

Servings: 4
Ingredients:
4 cups apple cider (pasteurized)
2 cups cranberry juice (diet)
2 quarts 7UP Diet
Half teaspoon cinnamon
Nutmeg (1/2 teaspoon)
1/2 teaspoon cloves, ground
1 cinnamon stick (optional)
Directions:

In a large pot, combine all Ingredients: and simmer until lukewarm.
Serve and enjoy.

Nutritional value:
- Energy value: 133 Kcal
- Protein: 0g
- Carbohydrates: 33 g
- Fiber: 0 g
- Sugar: 22g
- Sodium: 5 mg
- Fat: 0 g
- Of which:
- - Saturated: 0 g
- - Monounsaturated: 0 g
- - Polyunsaturated: 0 g
- - Cholesterol: 0 mg

178. LEMON COOLER

Servings: 4
Ingredients:
4 ice cubes, large
A quarter cup of lemon juice
A quarter cup of half and half cream
3 teaspoons sugar
Directions:
In a blender, combine all ingredients.
Set the blender on ice/crush and blend for 30 seconds to a minute, or until the ice is well crushed and the slush has reached the desired consistency.
Pour into a glass and, if desired, garnish with a slice of lemon.

Nutritional value:
- Energy value: 130 Kcal
- Protein: 1g
- Carbohydrates: 22 g
- Fiber: 0 g
- Sugar: 10g
- Sodium: 115mg
- Fat:4 g
- Of which:
- - Saturated: 2 g
- - Monounsaturated: g1
- - Polyunsaturated: 1 g
- - Cholesterol: 5mg

179. LEMON SMOOTHIE

Servings: 4
Ingredients:
4 cups apple cider (pasteurized)
2 cups cranberry juice (diet)
2 quarts 7UP® Diet
1/2 teaspoon cinnamon
Nutmeg (1/2 teaspoon)
1/2 teaspoon cloves, ground
1 cinnamon stick (optional)
Directions:
In a large Crock-Pot®, combine all Ingredients: and heat over low heat until lukewarm.
Serve and enjoy.

Nutritional value:
- Energy value: 153 Kcal
- Protein: 7 g

- Carbohydrates: 16 g
- Fiber: 7 g
- Sugar: 5 g
- Sodium: 2 g
- Fat: 13 g
- Of which:
- - Saturated: 4 g
- - Monounsaturated: 6 g
- - Polyunsaturated: 2 g
- Cholesterol: 115 mg

180.   LEMONADE OR LIMEADE BASE

Servings: 3
Ingredients:
2 1/2 cups liquid
1-1 / 4 cup sugar or sugar substitute (Splenda)
1/2 teaspoon lemon or lime zest, finely grated
1-1 / 4 cup freshly squeezed lime or lemon juice
Ice cubes
Directions:
Stir water and sugar or sugar substitute in a medium saucepan over medium heat until sugar dissolves. Remove from heat and let cool for 20 minutes. (Skip the heat if you are in a hurry). Instead, dissolve sugar in warm water and continue with step 2).
Stir citrus zest and juice into the sugar mixture. Fill a jar or pitcher half full with the mixture, cover and chill. Lasts up to 3 days in the refrigerator.
In ice-filled glasses, combine 3 ounces of base and 3 ounces of water for each glass of lemonade or limeade. To enjoy, stir and sip slowly. Freeze leftover base in ice cube trays and use in place of ice in drinks.

Nutritional value:
- Energy value: 192 Kcal
- Protein: 19 g
- Carbohydrates: 15 g
- Fiber: 7 g
- Sugar: 3 g
- Sodium: 3 g
- Fat: 10 g
- Of which:
- - Saturated: 5 g
- - Monounsaturated: 3 g
- - Polyunsaturated: 1 g
- - Cholesterol: 127 mg

181.   LEMON AND BLUEBERRY PROTEIN DRINK LEMONADE

Servings: 4
Ingredients:
Lemonade, 1 oz. LiquaCelTM Protein Supplement
Cranberry juice cocktail (2 oz.)
Sparkling water, 2 oz.
1 lime wedge
Directions:
Combine liquid protein, cranberry juice and ice in a blender and blend until smooth. With a spoon, blend well together.
Add 2 ounces of sparkling mineral water to the mixture (or to taste). Serve with a lime wedge as a garnish.

Nutritional value:
- Energy value: 175 Kcal
- Protein: 13 g
- Carbohydrates: 11 g

- Fiber: 3 g
- Sugar: 2 g
- Sodium: 3 g
- Fat: 11 g
- Of which:
- - Saturated: 3 g
- - Monounsaturated: 5 g
- - Polyunsaturated: 2 g
- - Cholesterol: 87 mg

182.   MAPLE APPLE DELIGHT PROTEIN DRINK

Servings: 1
Ingredients:
Nova Source kidney formula, 1/2 cup
Maple syrup (two teaspoons)
1 tablespoon butter (apple)
Directions:
In a blender, combine all Ingredients: and blend until smooth.
Chill before serving.

Nutritional value:
- Energy value: 120 Kcal
- Protein: 0 g
- Carbohydrates: 30 g
- Fiber: 0g
- Sugar: 29 g
- Sodium: 35mg
- Fat: 0g
- Of which:
- - Saturated: 0 g
- - Monounsaturated:0 g
- - Polyunsaturated: 0g
- - Cholesterol: 0 mg

183.   MIXED BERRY PROTEIN SHAKE

Servings: 4
Ingredients:
4 ounces ice water
1 cup mixed berries, fresh or frozen
2 ice cubes
1 teaspoon Crystal Light berry-flavored liquid flavor-intensifier drops
Whipped cream topping (1/2 cup)
Whey protein powder (two scoops)
Directions:
Add water, frozen berries, ice cubes and liquid flavor enhancer drops to a blender. Blend until muddy and well combined.
Blend the whipped topping well.
Add a little protein powder. Blend well.
Divide mixture into two servings and eat one right away, or freeze and eat later.

Nutritional value:
- Energy value: 110Kcal
- Protein: 12g
- Carbohydrates: 13 g
- Fiber: 5 g
- Sugar: 7g
- Sodium: 220mg
- Fat: 2 g
- Of which:
- - Saturated: 0g
- - Monounsaturated: 0 g

- Polyunsaturated: 2 g
- Cholesterol: 10mg

184. PINEAPPLE AND MINT FLAVORED WATER

Servings: 6
Ingredients:
1 cup pineapple (fresh)
12 mint leaves, new
10 liters of water
Directions:
Pineapple cut into cubes.
Mint leaves should be chopped.
In a pitcher, combine all ingredients.
Refrigerate for at least 24 hours before serving.

Nutritional value:
- Energy value: 78Kcal
- Protein: 1g
- Carbohydrates:22 g
- Fiber: 2g
- Sugar: 16g
- Sodium: 5mg
- Fat: 1 g
- Of which:
- - Saturated: 0g
- - Monounsaturated: 0 g
- - Polyunsaturated: 1 g
- - Cholesterol: 0mg

185. PROTEIN-RICH PEACH FRUIT SMOOTHIE

Servings: 1
Ingredients:
Half a cup of ice
2 teaspoons Just Whites® (powdered egg whites)
3/4 cup new peaches
1 teaspoon sugar
Directions:
Blend peaches until smooth in a blender.
Blend remaining Ingredients: until completely smooth.

Nutritional value:
- Energy value: 153 Kcal
- Protein: 7 g
- Carbohydrates: 16 g
- Fiber: 7 g
- Sugar: 5 g
- Sodium: 2 g
- Fat: 13 g
- Of which:
- - Saturated: 4 g
- - Monounsaturated: 6 g
- - Polyunsaturated: 2 g
- - Cholesterol: 115 mg

186. ORANGE AND PINEAPPLE SORBET PUNCH

Servings: 4
Ingredients:
1 cup pineapple (orange) juice.
1/2 gallon of sherbet of your favorite flavor
2-liter bottle of chilled lemon-lime soda with diet carbonated water.
Directions:
In a punch bowl, combine juice and sorbet.
Fill the remaining space in the bowl with lemon-lime soda.

Nutritional value:
- Energy value: 192 Kcal
- Protein: 19 g
- Carbohydrates: 15 g
- Fiber: 7 g
- Sugar: 3 g
- Sodium: 3 g
- Fat: 10 g
- Of which:
- - Saturated: 5 g
- - Monounsaturated: 3 g
- - Polyunsaturated: 1 g
- - Cholesterol: 127 mg

187. MARTHA'S COFFEE FRAPPÉ

Servings: 2
Ingredients:
1/3 cup of very cold coffee
A quarter cup of almond milk
Sugar (1-2 teaspoons)
1 tablespoon of chocolate syrup
Half a cup of ice cubes
Directions:
To make a smooth slushie, combine all ingredients in a blender and blend until smooth.
Pour immediately into a tall glass and serve.

Nutritional value:
- Energy value: 97 Kcal
- Protein: 1g
- Carbohydrates: 21 g
- Fiber: 1g
- Sugar: 15g
- Sodium: 53mg
- Fat: 1g
- Of which:
- - Saturated: 1 g
- - Monounsaturated: 0 g
- - Polyunsaturated: 0g
- - Cholesterol: 0mg

RENAL PLAN

WEEK Nº. 1

Monday	Breakfast: • 2 Cubes of gelatin energy with high protein content Snack: • 2 logs of peanut butter and jellied celery Lunch: • 9 oz of Jamaican chicken • 3½ oz of creamy orzo and vegetables • 1 glass of lemonade Snack: • 1¾ oz of popcorn ball Dinner: • Ground beef and vegetable dinner in the foil packet
Tuesday	Breakfast: • 1 soup spoonful of hot Multicereal cereal Snack: • 2 logs of peanut butter and jellied celery Lunch: • Lemon-garlic chicken with quinoa and orzo • 1 glass of lemonade Snack: • 1 protein Booster Blueberry Muffin Dinner: • Chicken with lemon and cilantro • Natural juice without sugar
Wednesday	Breakfast: • Maple and honey nut mix. Snack: • A couple of cream cheese thumbprint crackers. Lunch: • 9 oz of roasted rosemary vegetables and chicken. • 1 fruit smoothie Snack: • 1 Jackie's Cornbread Muffins Dinner: • Roasted turkey breast with salt-free herb seasoning.
Thursday	Breakfast: • 3 German pancakes • 1 fresh orange juice Snack: • 1 egg in a hole Lunch: • 10¾ oz of the pickled okra. • A couple of omelets of mushrooms and red bell pepper • 1 glass of lemon set with mint Snack: • 1 egg muffin Dinner:

	<ul><li>3 slices of pumpkin bread and blueberries</li><li>1 glass of unsweetened natural juice</li></ul>
Friday	Breakfast:<ul><li>9 oz of oatmeal and blueberry cookies.</li></ul>Snack:<ul><li>One puffed baked pancake</li></ul>Lunch:<ul><li>Pakoda</li><li>1 glass of natural juice</li></ul>Snack:<ul><li>1 cup with dried fruit</li></ul>Dinner:<ul><li>2 slices of apple and zucchini bread.</li><li>1 protein shake</li></ul>
Saturday	Breakfast:<ul><li>4 oatmeal bars with unbaked peanuts.</li></ul>Snack:<ul><li>3½ oz of poppy krunch.</li></ul>Lunch:<ul><li>10 oz of lemonade wings</li><li>2 corn tortillas</li><li>1 glass of natural juice without sugar.</li></ul>Snack:<ul><li>1 low-phosphorus sugar candy.</li></ul>Dinner:<ul><li>3 slices of lemon bread and berries.</li><li>1 glass of natural juice without sugar.</li></ul>
Sunday	Breakfast:<ul><li>1 bagel with cream cheese, tomato and onion.</li></ul>Snack:<ul><li>1 cup frozen fruit delight</li></ul>Lunch:<ul><li>7 oz of spaghetti frittata with basil.</li><li>A lumpia</li><li>1 glass of lemonade</li></ul>Snack:<ul><li>1 large glass of protein drinkMaple Apple Delight.</li></ul>Dinner:<ul><li>2 slices of toasted bread, spread with lemon pepper hummus.</li><li>Unsweetened natural juice</li></ul>

WEEK Nº. 2

Monday:	Breakfast: • 2 festive morning French toast. Snack: • 3½ oz of popcorn Lunch: • 3½ oz of Lemon rice with vegetables. • 9 oz of Indian Curry Chicken • 1 glass of Party Punch Snack: • 1¾ oz of Popcorn. Dinner: • French toast with hummus • Natural juice without sugar
Tuesday	Breakfast: • 1 egg and sausage breakfast sandwich. Snack: • 1 protein-boosting blueberry muffin Lunch: • 3½ oz of egg pockets • 3½–7 oz of Italian Meatballs • 1 glass of Lemon Cooler Snack: • Fruit smoothie Dinner: • Pineapple and sweet onion salsa with tortilla chips.
Wednesday	Breakfast: • Festive scrambled eggs Snack: • 1 Jackie's cornbread muffin. Lunch: • 3 Celery sticks with hummus and red bell pepper. • 2 Hula Meatballs • 1 Glass of lemon-cranberry protein drink lemonade Snack: • 1 Mixed berry protein shake. Dinner: • A cream cheese dip with mint jelly.
Thursday	Breakfast: • 2 heavenly Jalas Snack: • Egg muffin Lunch: • 9 oz of feta pasta with chicken and asparagus. • 1 glass of lemonade Snack: • 1 protein-rich peach fruit smoothie. Dinner: • A cream cheese dip with mint jelly.
Friday	Breakfast: • 9 oz of festive scrambled eggs.

	• A couple of French toast Snack: • 1 cup of hot Wassail Lunch: • 9 oz of rice and Louisiana Style Stewed Chicken. • 1 Glass of pineapple and mint flavored water Snack: • Martha's Coffee Frappé Dinner: • 3 Slices of Pumpkin Blueberry Bread • 1 Glass of unsweetened natural juice
Saturday	Breakfast: • 1 Soup cup of Hot Multicereal cereal. Snack: • 1 cup of dried fruit Lunch: • 10¾ oz of skillet chicken with green beans and potatoes. • 1 Glass of mint lemonade • 2 Grilled Corn Pancakes with Cheese (Arepas) Snack: • A couple of oatmeal cookies Dinner: • Chicken with lemon and cilantro • Natural juice without sugar
Sunday	Breakfast: • 2 German pancakes • 1 Natural juice without sugar Snack: • 1 Protein-boosting blueberry muffin Lunch: • 9 oz of turkey meatloaf • 1 Glass of unsweetened natural juice • 3½ oz of blueberry and roasted garlic risotto Snack: • 1¾ oz of popcorn Dinner: • Ground beef and vegetable dinner in the foil packet.

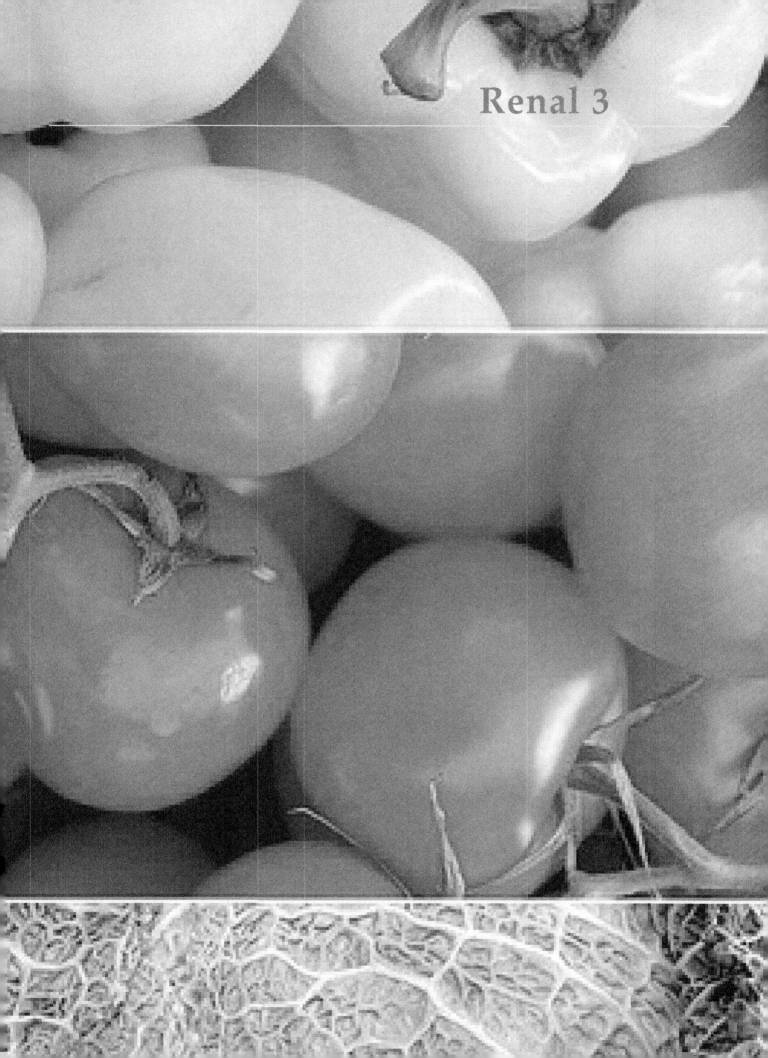

INTRODUCTION

The general objective of this book is to provide the reader and patients with renal diseases, a balanced diet plan that will allow them to reduce the symptoms of this pathology.

In the case of healthy people, this eating plan will also help them to prevent these and other diseases of the organism. This prevention also involves making drastic changes in diet and physical activities to reduce sedentary lifestyle, a silent enemy for our body and also the cause of degenerative diseases.

Food changes

These dietary changes have a direct impact on the choice of foods, for which the following is recommended:

- Instead of choosing foods high in fat, choose those low in fat. Example: yogurt, 1% skim milk, margarine, etc.
- Prefer fresh fruits and vegetables as snacks and refreshments.
- Prepare vegetarian meals several times a week
- Consume fruits as dessert
- When buying meat, prefer lean cuts: center, loin, sirloin, tenderloin, leg and eliminate all visible fat.
- Avoid fried foods. Use other healthier cooking options, prefer steamed food, stews, grills.
- Season meats with natural spices. Thyme, paprika, turmeric or homemade tomato sauce, garlic, oregano, basil.
- Drastically reduce salt intake.
- Include a diet rich in calcium, to contribute to the strengthening of bones. Among the lowest fat and calorie sources of calcium are soy milk and low-fat yogurt. Calcium is also present in some green leafy vegetables, broccoli, sardines with bones or canned sardines and salmon.
- Choose healthy carbohydrates. Carbohydrates include fiber, starch and sugar. Natural sugar is present in some fruits and vegetables. Avoid regular consumption of cakes, soft drinks, cookies, ice cream. Replace starch with cereals, whole-grain bread, whole grain pasta and rice, and legumes.

Changes in physical activities

Physical activity generates great health benefits. The list is extensive, some of those benefits are:

- Helping you feel, look and sleep better.
- Helps you stay in shape to cope with all your daily activities.
- Improves bone density and muscle strength, facilitating flexibility and balance.
- It reduces the risk of disease.
- Physical activity also contributes to lower triglycerides and increases HDL cholesterol or good cholesterol in the blood.
- Helps lower blood pressure
- It lowers blood glucose and makes the body more sensitive to insulin.

Now that you know the benefits of daily physical activity, it is convenient to establish a weekly goal that is achievable, for this it is necessary:

- Make an advance planning of the exercise routine. Set goals for the achievement of these objectives. However, it is advisable that before complying with a rigorous physical activity consult your doctor and get his approval as an endorsement to advance the level of physical activities.
- Choose activities that you enjoy: walking, aerobics, swimming, dance therapy, etc.
- Choose types of physical activities that are of moderate intensity, such as brisk walking.
- Work on each of the goals you set for yourself, dividing those activities into several days of the week. For example, if in one week you did more than 60 minutes of activities, work gradually to increase the time of physical activities, a good rule is to increase no more than 30 minutes a day. Example:

Week 1:	Walk 60 minutes per week. This equals 12 minutes in 5 days.
Week 2:	Walk 90 minutes per week, or 18 minutes in 5 days.
Week 3:	Walk 120 minutes per week, that is, 24 minutes per 5 days.
Week 4:	Walk 150 minutes per week, that is, 30 minutes in 5 days.

Hence, the importance of weekly planning. Plan in advance the time you will spend being active, don't just wait for that activity to happen. Instead, make it happen!

There are even times when we have the opportunity to make a more active decision, some of these moments occur spontaneously and often the activity will be brief. However, the sum of all these moments could make all the difference in starting to change your physical activity habits.

In this book, we not only want you to be able to stick to a healthy eating plan but also to a program that will provide holistic benefits to your body. Remember, the success of a healthy and balanced diet must be combined with daily physical activity.

Physical activity prevention

The smart way to be active is to be active safely. To do this, it is important to prevent some of these problems:

- **Prevent muscle soreness or cramps:** for this, it is necessary to gradually increase the intensity of the physical exercise routine in frequency, intensity and in time duration. When starting physical activity make sure you are sufficiently hydrated and warm up before and after the activity.

- **Maintain safety while stretching your muscles:** Stretching is one of the best options to prevent muscle aches, cramps or other ailments. This will also help you feel more relaxed. Here is the best way to stretch:

  - Perform a short warm-up prior to stretching.
  - Move slowly until you feel the muscles stretching.
  - Hold the stretch steady for 15 to 30 minutes.
  - Relax, repeat again 3 to 5 times.
  - Be careful to stretch both sides of the body. It is imperative to maintain balance.
  - Stretch within your own limits. This is not a competition.
  - Do not hold your breath. On the contrary, breathe slowly and naturally.
  - Always stay in control. Sudden and unstable movements can lead to injury.
  - If you have any pain, do not do any type of stretching.
  - If a particular stretch causes you any pain. Stop and give it some attention.
  - In case of injury or you are unable to move the injured area, or if there is any immediate severe swelling, consult your physician.

BREAKFAST:

188. ZUCCHINI MUFFINS

Servings: 4
Ingredients:
3 cups all-purpose white flour
3/4 cups Splenda granulated sugar or sweetener
1-1/2 teaspoons pumpkin pie spice
1-1/2 teaspoons baking soda
1 teaspoon salt
4 eggs
2 cups shredded zucchini
3/4 cup honey
1/3 cup oil
1/3 cup unsweetened applesauce
2 tablespoons lemon juice
1 teaspoon vanilla extract
Directions:
Preheat oven to 375°F.
In a large bowl, whisk together flour, sugar, pumpkin pie spice, baking soda and salt.
In a medium bowl, beat the eggs lightly. Add the zucchini, honey, oil, applesauce, lemon juice and vanilla.
Stir the liquid mixture into the flour combination until the flour is moistened.
Grease muffin tins or use baking paper. Fill each cup 3/4 full.
Bake for 15 to 20 minutes or until the toothpick is soft.

Nutritional value:
• Energy value: 175 Kcal
• Protein: 13 g
• Carbohydrates: 11 g
• Fiber: 3 g
• Sugar: 2 g
• Sodium: 3 g
• Fat: 11 g
• Of which:
• - Saturated: 3 g
• - Monounsaturated: 5 g
• - Polyunsaturated: 2 g
- Cholesterol: 87 mg

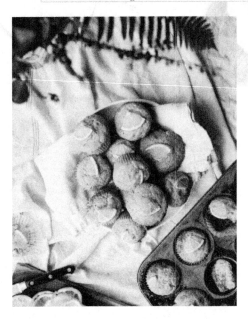

189. SUPER SIMPLE BAKED PANCAKE

Servings: 2
Ingredients:
2 large eggs
half a cup of milk
Half cup of white flour for all causes
1/4 teaspoon salt
1/8 teaspoon nutmeg
1 tablespoon vegetable oil
Directions:
Preheat oven to 450°F.
Beat the eggs and milk in a medium bowl with a wire whisk or electric mixer.
Whisk in the flour, salt and nutmeg until blended (small lumps of flour remaining in the batter are okay).
Pour the oil directly into a 9" ovenproof skillet or pie pan and place the area in the preheated oven for 5 minutes to heat the oil.
Carefully pour the batter into the skillet and bake exposed for 18 to 20 minutes. (Avoid turning on the oven door until the pancake is over-iced and crisp around the edges. The middle may brown while cooking).
Cut into four wedges and serve with pancake syrup or fruit spread.

Nutritional value:
• Energy value: 153 Kcal
• Protein: 7 g
• Carbohydrates: 16 g
• Fiber: 7 g
• Sugar: 5 g
• Sodium: 2 g
• Fat: 13 g
• Of which:
• - Saturated: 4 g
• - Monounsaturated: 6 g
• - Polyunsaturated: 2 g
• - Cholesterol: 115 mg

190. MAPLE PANCAKES

Servings: 2
Ingredients:
1 cup plain flour
1 tablespoon granulated sugar
2 teaspoons baking powder
1/8 teaspoon salt
2 large egg whites
1 cup 1% skim milk
2 tablespoons canola oil
1 tablespoon maple extract
Directions:
In a medium bowl, integrate the flour, sugar, baking powder and salt. Make a well in the center of the dry mixture. Set aside.
In a large bowl, integrate egg whites, milk, oil and maple extract.
Add the egg mixture to the dry mixture. Stir until moistened (batter should be lumpy).

To make 4" pancakes, pour about 1/4 cup batter onto a lightly greased hot griddle or heavy skillet.

Cook over medium heat for about 2 minutes on each side or until pancakes are golden brown. Flip the pancake as long as it has a bubbly floor and the edges are barely dry. To keep the pancakes light and fluffy, flip them as soon as possible and avoid pressing with a spatula.

Nutritional value:
- Energy value: 192 Kcal
- Protein: 19 g
- Carbohydrates: 15 g
- Fiber: 7 g
- Sugar: 3 g
- Sodium: 3 g
- Fat: 10 g
- Of which:
- - Saturated: 5 g
- - Monounsaturated: 3 g
- - Polyunsaturated: 1 g
- - Cholesterol: 127 mg

191.   STUFFED FRENCH TOAST

Servings: 5
Ingredients:
8 oz. Cream cheese
1 lb. loaf of French bread from the day before
8 tablespoons gelatin, any flavor
6 large eggs
1 cup 1% low-fat milk
1 teaspoon vanilla extract
Directions:
Cut loaf of bread into sixteen slices.
Spread 1 tablespoon cream cheese on each slice of bread. Top with 1 tablespoon gelatin and add a slice of bread to make a sandwich.
Repeat until 8 sandwiches are prepared.
Spray a 9 "x 13" baking dish with nonstick cooking spray and near the 8 sandwiches inside the dish.
Beat the eggs and then mix with the milk and vanilla extract. Pour over the bread slices, turning to coat the slices lightly. Cover and refrigerate in one day.
Preheat oven to 350°F. Cover pan with foil and bake for 1 hour. For the last five minutes of baking, remove the foil to brown the pinnacle.

Nutritional value:
- Energy value: 135 Kcal
- Protein: 7 g
- Carbohydrates: 6 g
- Fiber: 5 g
- Sugar: 4 g
- Sodium: 5 g
- Fat: 10 g
- Of which:
- - Saturated: 5 g
- - Monounsaturated: 3 g
- - Polyunsaturated: 1 g
- - Cholesterol: 167 mg

192.   BLUEBERRIES IN THE SNOW

Servings: 5
Ingredients:
1 cup cherry cranberry juice
12 ounces of clean cranberries

2 packages Knox unflavored gelatin
2 cups granulated sugar
1 cup whipped pineapple, canned in juice
8 oz cream cheese
3 cups Reddi-Wip whipped topping.
Directions:
In a medium saucepan, bring cran-cherry juice to a boil.
Add cranberries and return to a boil, after which reduce heat to medium. Cook until berries are soft, about 10 to 12 minutes.
Remove the pan from the heat. Stir in gelatin and 1-1/four cups sugar. Stir until sugar dissolves. Let cool, approximately 30 minutes.
Add tired pineapple to cranberry combination. Mix well. Pour the aggregate right into a nine "x thirteen" pan or for a man or woman servings, pour 1/3 cup of the blueberry mixture into dessert glasses. Chill until set, about 1 hour.
Let the cream cheese melt, about 30 minutes.
Prepare topping in a large bowl by mixing the final 3/4 cup sugar and softened cream cheese with a hand mixer. Gently fold into the whipped topping.
Spread the topping gently over the frozen blueberry addition in a pan or place 1/4 cup on top of each man or woman serving. Refrigerate to set.

Nutritional value:
- Energy value: 173 Kcal
- Protein: 8 g
- Carbohydrates: 4 g
- Fiber: 4 g
- Sugar: 2 g
- Sodium: 4 g
- Fat: 12 g
- Of which:
- - Saturated: 3 g
- - Monounsaturated: 5 g
- - Polyunsaturated: 4 g
- - Cholesterol: 149 mg

193.   APPLE BARS

Servings: 4
Ingredients:
2 medium apples
3/4 cup unsalted butter
1 cup granulated sugar
1 cup sour cream
1 teaspoon vanilla extract
1 teaspoon baking soda
1/2 teaspoon salt
2 cups whole wheat flour
1/2 cup brown sugar
1 teaspoon cinnamon
2 tablespoons milk
1 cup powdered sugar
Directions:
Preheat oven to 350°F.
Peel and chop the apples.
Beat in half cup butter and granulated sugar or granulated sugar substitute.
Add sour cream, vanilla, baking soda, salt and flour. Stir to blend; stir in chopped apples.
Pour batter into a greased nine "x thirteen" baking pan.
In a small bowl, disintegrate 2 tablespoons of softened butter, brown sugar and cinnamon together. Sprinkle over the pinnacle of dough.
Bake for 35 to 40 minutes. Let cool absolutely.
To make the glaze, combine 2 tablespoons of melted butter, milk (or milk substitute) and powdered sugar. Drizzle over the top and cut the dessert into 18 bars.

Nutritional value:
- Energy value: 168 Kcal
- Protein: 13 g
- Carbohydrates: 12 g
- Fiber: 4 g
- Sugar: 2 g
- Sodium: 2 g
- Fat: 15 g
- Of which:
- - Saturated: 5 g
- - Monounsaturated: 4 g
- - Polyunsaturated: 5 g
- - Cholesterol: 153 mg

194. BLUEBERRY AND PEACH CRISP

Servings: 4
Ingredients:
7 medium peaches
1 cup blueberries
1/4 cup granulated sugar
1 tablespoon lemon juice
3/4 cup flour for all motifs
3/4 cup packed brown sugar
1/2 cup butter
Directions:
Preheat oven to 375°F.
Core and cut peaches into 3/4 slices.
Spray a 12 "x nine" baking dish with cooking spray. Arrange peach slices and blueberries in a dish.
Sprinkle sugar and lemon juice over the fruit.
Mix flour and brown sugar in a bowl. With two knives or a pastry blender, reduce the butter to the flour and sugar combination until crumbly. Sprinkle the crumbs over the fruit.
Bake for 45 minutes or longer until the fruit is soft and crumbs are golden brown.
Serve warm at room temperature.

Nutritional value:
- Energy value: 192 Kcal
- Protein: 19 g
- Carbohydrates: 15 g
- Fiber: 7 g
- Sugar: 3 g

- Sodium: 3 g
- Fat: 10 g
- Of which:
- - Saturated: 5 g
- - Monounsaturated: 3 g
- - Polyunsaturated: 1 g
- Cholesterol: 127 mg

195. RICE PUDDING (ARROZ CON LECHE)

Servings: 4
Ingredients:
1 cup uncooked white rice
2 cups of unsweetened almond milk
2 tablespoons raisins
1/4 cup granulated sugar
1/4 teaspoon cinnamon
1 teaspoon vanilla extract
Directions:
Rinse rice with tap water, then drain.
Add rice and 1 cup water to a medium saucepan. Bring to a boil, cover with a lid and cook dinner for 10 minutes.
Remove the lid and add the almond milk and raisins. Cover again and boil for 10 minutes or until rice is cooked through. (The rice will have a thick consistency; not all the liquid will evaporate).
When the rice is done, remove from the heat and mix with the sugar (or sugar alternative), cinnamon and vanilla. Mix well and serve hot. Refrigerate any leftovers.

Nutritional value:
- Energy value: 175 Kcal
- Protein: 13 g
- Carbohydrates: 11 g
- Fiber: 3 g
- Sugar: 2 g
- Sodium: 3 g
- Fat: 11 g
- Of which:
- - Saturated: 3 g
- - Monounsaturated: 5 g
- - Polyunsaturated: 2 g
- Cholesterol: 87 mg

Brunch:

196. TOMATO JAR APPETIZER

Servings: 5
Ingredients:
4 Roma tomatoes, strong
1 tablespoon extra-virgin olive oil
1 teaspoon freshly ground black pepper
1 teaspoon garlic powder
1 teaspoon herb seasoning mix (unsalted)
15 ounces canned chickpeas
Half a lemon
1 teaspoon vinegar (red wine)
8 mint leaves, new
Directions:
To make "boats," cut tomatoes in half and discard flesh.
Drizzle 1/2 tablespoon olive oil, 1/2 teaspoon pepper, 1/2 teaspoon garlic powder and 1/2 teaspoon salt-free seasoning into the tomato boats.
Chickpeas should be rinsed and drained. Combine chickpeas, remaining olive oil, spices, juice of 1/2 lemon and vinegar in a mixing bowl. Combine all ingredients:
Fill the tomato cups halfway with the chickpea mixture. Serve with a mint leaf as a garnish.
Refrigerate until ready to eat.

Nutritional value:	
•	Energy value: 60 Kcal
•	Protein: 1g
•	Carbohydrates: 8 g
•	Fiber: 1g
•	Sugar: 0 g
•	Sodium: 261mg
•	Fat: 2g
•	Of which:
•	- Saturated: 0g
•	- Monounsaturated: 2 g
•	- Polyunsaturated: 0 g
Cholesterol: 0mg	

197. SHRIMP STUFFED EGGS

Servings: 3
Ingredients:
6 large hard-boiled eggs
1/2 cup shrimp (cooked)
Mustard (1/2 teaspoon)
1 1/2 teaspoon mayonnaise
1/4 teaspoon lemon juice
1 teaspoon cayenne pepper
Directions:
Cooked eggs should be cut in half lengthwise. Carefully remove the yolks and place them on a plate.
Finely chop the shrimp and combine with the mustard, mayonnaise, lemon juice and pepper in the egg yolks. Mix until all ingredients are well blended.
Fill half of an egg white with the shrimp and yolk mixture.

Nutritional value:	
•	Energy value: 132 Kcal
•	Protein: 10g
•	Carbohydrates: 6 g
•	Fiber: 1g
•	Sugar: 1g
•	Sodium: 360mg
•	Fat: 7g
•	Of which:
•	- Saturated: 2g
•	- Monounsaturated: 3 g
•	- Polyunsaturated: 2 g
- Cholesterol: 243 mg	

198. INDIVIDUAL FRITTATAS

Servings: 4
Ingredients:
1 pound of frozen hash brown potatoes
2 ounces cooked lean ham
2 tablespoons pink bell pepper
2 tablespoons inexperienced bell pepper
2 tablespoons onion
4 huge eggs
1 tablespoon 1% low-fat milk
1/8 teaspoon black pepper
1/2 cup shredded low-fat cheddar cheese
Directions:
Soak hash brown potatoes in a large bowl of water for four hours. Drain, rinse and squeeze out excess water. (Skip this step if low potassium is not desired).
Preheat oven to 375°F. Coat eight muffin tin holes with cooking spray.
Using a 1/3 cup measure, place potato croquettes in muffin tins and press the potato into the back and up the edges of each muffin. Spray the potato croquettes with cooking spray. Place within the oven and bake dinner for 15 minutes and discard from oven. Reduce oven temperature to 350°F.
Finely chop the ham, peppers and onion. Whisk eggs and milk collectively in a medium bowl; season with black pepper. Add ham, peppers, onion and cheese to the egg combination and combine.
Partly press baked hash browns down firmly with a spoon so that the potatoes cover the bottom and sides of each hollow muffin. Pour 1/4 cup of the egg mixture into the center of the eight muffin tins. Return the pan to the oven and bake until the potatoes are crisp and golden brown and the egg mixture is firm, about 15 to twenty minutes.
Remove the muffin pan from the oven and let stand approximately five minutes before serving.

Nutritional value:	
•	Energy value: 192 Kcal
•	Protein: 19 g
•	Carbohydrates: 15 g
•	Fiber: 7 g
•	Sugar: 3 g
•	Sodium: 3 g
•	Fat: 10 g
•	Of which:
•	- Saturated: 5 g
•	- Monounsaturated: 3 g
•	- Polyunsaturated: 1 g
•	- Cholesterol: 127 mg

199. PITA POCKETS ROLL

Servings: 4
Ingredients:
2 tablespoons olive oil
1 medium onion
2 cups of mushrooms

1 medium red bell pepper
1/2 cup flat-leaf parsley 1 pound lean ground beef
1 tablespoon Worcestershire sauce
1 tablespoon browning and seasoning cooking sauce
1/2 teaspoon black pepper
6 pieces pita bread

Directions:
Slice onion and mushrooms; cut bell pepper into thin strips. Chop the parsley.
Heat the olive oil in a large skillet over medium-high heat.
Add onion, bell pepper and mushrooms. Sauté until vegetables are tender, about 6 minutes. Remove vegetables to a plate.
Add the meat to the skillet and cook until no trace of pink remains 5 to 6 minutes. Spoon off the fat.
Add Worcestershire sauce, Kitchen Bouquet Sauce and black pepper; stir and cook 1 to 2 minutes.
Add vegetables to meat and stir to combine.
Stir in parsley and cook until heated through. Remove from heat.
Hot Pitas. Cut a 2" strip from the side of each pita and open it.
Stuff each pita with the meat and vegetable mixture.

> **Nutritional value:**
> - Energy value: 267 Kcal
> - Protein: 15g
> - Carbohydrates: 56 g
> - Fiber: 8g
> - Sugar: 4g
> - Sodium: 336mg
> - Fat: 4g
> - Of which:
> - - Saturated: 2 g
> - - Monounsaturated:1 g
> - - Polyunsaturated: 1g
> - Cholesterol: 10 mg

200.   TORTILLA WRAPS

Servings: 1
Ingredients:
Carrots, 2 teaspoons
2 tablespoons pepper (green)
Cucumber, 1/3 cup
2/3 cup cooked chicken, unsalted
2 flour tortillas, 6" in diameter
4 tablespoons cream cheese (whipped)
One-quarter teaspoon garlic powder
One-quarter teaspoon onion powder
One-third cup broccoli slaw mix.

Directions:
Carrots should be shredded, green bell pepper and cucumber chopped and chicken shredded.
Cream cheese with garlic and onion powder.
Half of the mixture should be spread on each tortilla.
Add vegetables and chicken.
Refrigerate or serve directly after rolling the wrap.

> **Nutritional value:**
> - - Energy value: 175 Kcal
> - - Protein: 13 g
> - - Carbohydrates: 11 g
> - - Fiber: 3 g
> - - Sugar: 2 g
> - - Sodium: 3 g
> - - Fat: 11 g
> - - Of which:

> - - Saturated: 3 g
> - - Monounsaturated: 5 g
> - - Polyunsaturated: 2 g
> - Cholesterol: 87 mg

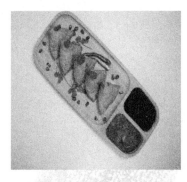

201.   SAMOSA

Servings: 1
Ingredients:
1 tablespoon onion
2 tablespoons coriander 1 teaspoon ginger root
1/2 cup peas, frozen
3 tablespoons canola oil plus frying oil
1 tablespoon coriander powder
1/4 teaspoon cayenne pepper
1 teaspoon garam masala (garam masala)
1 pound ground beef
24 spring roll cakes (1 package)
2 teaspoons all-purpose white flour
2 teaspoons distilled water

Directions:
Finely chop onion, ginger root and cilantro. Thaw the frozen green peas outside.
In a large skillet, heat 3 tablespoons of oil over medium heat.
Combine onion, ginger root, cilantro, bell pepper and Garam Masala in a mixing bowl.
Cook, stirring constantly, until ground beef is no longer pink. The fat should drain away.
Cook until the mixture is dry, then stir in the peas. Stir in the cilantro.
Create a thin paste with 1 tablespoon of flour and quite hot.
On a floured surface, roll out the puff pastry. Fold the dough over and place 2 tablespoons of the meat mixture in the middle. Using a paste of flour and water, seal the edges.
Fry the pastry in hot oil until golden brown.

> **Nutritional value:**
> - Energy value: 192 Kcal
> - Protein: 19 g
> - Carbohydrates: 15 g
> - Fiber: 7 g
> - Sugar: 3 g
> - Sodium: 3 g
> - Fat: 10 g
> - Of which:
> - - Saturated: 5 g
> - - Monounsaturated: 3 g
> - - Polyunsaturated: 1 g
> - - Cholesterol: 127 mg

SIDE DISHES AND snacks:

202. POPCORN WITH SUGAR AND SPICES

Servings: 5
Ingredients:
8 cups of popcorn (made with air).
2 tablespoons butter (unsalted)
2 teaspoons sugar
Half teaspoon cinnamon
A quarter teaspoon of nutmeg
Directions:
In a saucepan, heat the butter, sugar, cinnamon and nutmeg until the butter melts and the sugar dissolves. Microwave the Ingredients: in a microwave-safe bowl if desired. Make sure the butter does not smoke.
Drizzle the spiced butter mixture over the popcorn and stir to combine.
Serve immediately for best yield.

> **Nutritional value:**
> - Energy value: 153 Kcal
> - Protein: 7 g
> - Carbohydrates: 16 g
> - Fiber: 7 g
> - Sugar: 5 g
> - Sodium: 2 g
> - Fat: 13 g
> - Of which:
> - Saturated: 4 g
> - Monounsaturated: 6 g
> - Polyunsaturated: 2 g
> - Cholesterol: 115 mg

203. SOFT PRETZELS

Servings: 4
Ingredients:
2 cups of warm water
2 applications of dry active yeast
Four tablespoons canola oil
Five half cups white all-purpose flour (divided)
6 cups water
3 tablespoons baking soda
1/4 cup mustard
Directions:
Dissolve yeast in warm water and let stand for 10 minutes.
Add the canola oil and half of the flour. Stir until well blended. Add the final flour and knead for five minutes.
Cover and let the dough rest for 1 hour.
Divide the dough into 24 portions. Roll into 18" lengths and twist into a pretzel shape. Let push up for half an hour.
Preheat oven to 475°F.
Add baking soda to 6 cups of water in a large pot and bring to a boil.
Add pretzels to boiling water for 1 minute, then transfer to a baking sheet sprayed with nonstick cooking spray.
Bake for 12 minutes.
Serve each pretzel with 1/2 teaspoon mustard.

> **Nutritional value:**
> - Energy value: 380 Kcal
> - Protein: 10g
> - Carbohydrates:80 g

> - Fiber: 3g
> - Sugar: 3g
> - Sodium: 126mg
> - Fat: 3g
> - Of which:
> - Saturated: 1 g
> - Monounsaturated:1 g
> - Polyunsaturated: 1g
> - Cholesterol: 0 mg

204. SWEET POPCORN BALLS

Servings: 6
Ingredients:
16 cups of unsalted popcorn
2 cups Karo® dark corn syrup
2 cups sugar (brown)
1 liter of water
1 teaspoon vinegar
4 tablespoons butter (whipped)
Directions:
Pop the popcorn and place it in a large bowl. Set aside for later use.
In a saucepan, combine the syrup, brown sugar, water and vinegar. Cook, stirring continuously, over medium heat until the mixture comes to a boil. Cook for another 15-20 minutes over medium heat, stirring almost continuously. Cook until hardball is reached (until a small amount of mixture forms a hard ball when tested in very cold water).
Remove from the heat and quickly stir in the butter.
Slowly pour mixture over popped popcorn in a large mixing bowl, stirring constantly. With as little pressure as possible, roll into balls. Each popcorn ball should be wrapped in plastic wrap and stored in an airtight jar.

> **Nutritional value:**
> - Energy value:110 Kcal
> - Protein: 1g
> - Carbohydrates: 26 g
> - Fiber: 1g
> - Sugar: 18g
> - Sodium: 140mg
> - Fat: 1g
> - Of which:
> - Saturated: 0 g
> - Monounsaturated: 1 g
> - Polyunsaturated: 0 g
> - Cholesterol: 1 mg

205. SWEET AND SPICY TORTILLA CHIPS

Servings: 2

Ingredients:

1 tablespoon butter

1 teaspoon of sugar (brown)

1 /2 teaspoon chili powder, plant

1/4 teaspoon garlic powder

1/2 teaspoon cumin powder

1/4 teaspoon cayenne pepper, ground

6 flour tortillas, each 6" in diameter.

Directions:

Preheat oven to 425°F.

Coat a baking dish with cooking spray.

In a small bowl, melt butter and combine with brown sugar and spices.

Cut each tortilla into 8 wedges and place them in the baking dish in a single layer.

Coat the tortillas with the seasoning mixture using a pastry knife. Serve warm or cold, after baking for about 8 minutes until golden brown.

Store leftover chips in an airtight bag.

Nutritional value:

- Energy value: 192 Kcal
- Protein: 19 g
- Carbohydrates: 15 g
- Fiber: 7 g
- Sugar: 3 g
- Sodium: 3 g
- Fat: 10 g
- Of which:
- - Saturated: 5 g
- - Monounsaturated: 3 g
- - Polyunsaturated: 1 g
- - Cholesterol: 127 mg

VEGETARIAN DISHES:

206. FETTUCCINI ALFREDO

Servings: 4
Ingredients:
12 ounces of fettuccini, uncooked.
1 tablespoon olive oil
2 tablespoons unsalted butter
2 cloves garlic
3/4 cup red bell pepper
2 tablespoons all-purpose flour
1/3 cup white wine
1 cup low sodium chicken broth
1/2 cup half-and-half cream
2 teaspoons dried parsley flakes
1/4 teaspoon black pepper
1/4 cup grated Parmesan cheese
Directions:
Mince the garlic and slice the red bell pepper.
Cook the fettuccini according to the Directions: on the package, omitting the salt. Drain and set aside.
In a medium saucepan melt the butter and combine with the olive oil.
Add garlic and red bell pepper. Sauté for 1 to 2 minutes until vegetables are soft.
Slowly stir flour into skillet. Cook 1 minute until smooth.
Add wine gradually, stirring until smooth.
Add broth, cream, parsley and black pepper. Stir to combine.
Gradually stir in the Parmesan cheese. Reduce heat to low and cook for 5 to 7 minutes until mixture begins to simmer. Stir occasionally.
Toss the sauce with the drained fettuccini.

Nutritional value:
- Energy value: 175 Kcal
- Protein: 13 g
- Carbohydrates: 11 g
- Fiber: 3 g
- Sugar: 2 g
- Sodium: 3 g
- Fat: 11 g
- Of which:
- - Saturated: 3 g
- - Monounsaturated: 5 g
- - Polyunsaturated: 2 g
- - Cholesterol: 87 mg

207. TORTILLA ROLLS

Servings: 1
Ingredients:
1/2 cup spinach leaves, raw.
2 teaspoons shallots
2 tablespoons pimento cheese
3 ounces cooked turkey breast, raw
1/2 cup pineapple chunks
1/2 cup whipped cream cheese
2 flour tortillas, burrito size
1 teaspoon Mrs. Dash® original Mrs. Dash® herb seasoning blend.
Directions:
Finely chop spinach. Dice the onion, bell pepper and turkey breast.
Remove the pineapple and drain.
To top each tortilla, spread cream cheese on top. Mrs. Dash® herb seasoning, if desired.
In a bowl, combine the remaining ingredients.

Separate Ingredients into two parts. Half of each tortilla should be placed on top of the other and rolled up like a jelly roll.
Trim the ends of each roll and cut it into six pieces.

Nutritional value:
- Energy value: 153 Kcal
- Protein: 7 g
- Carbohydrates: 16 g
- Fiber: 7 g
- Sugar: 5 g
- Sodium: 2 g
- Fat: 13 g
- Of which:
- - Saturated: 4 g
- - Monounsaturated: 6 g
- - Polyunsaturated: 2 g
- - Cholesterol: 115 mg

208. RAW VEGETABLES AND SAUCE

Servings: 4
Ingredients:
A couple of teaspoons of Mrs. Dash's® herb seasoning for onions.
Half cup sour cream
2 stalks celery
1 cauliflower
1 bell pepper
Half a cucumber
A total of 8 radishes
Directions:
To merge flavors, combine Mrs. Dash's® herb relish with sour cream and chill for at least one hour.
Each celery stalk should be cut in half lengthwise and then cut into four sections.
Carrots should be cut in half lengthwise and then cut into four sections.
Remove the seeds from the bell pepper by cutting them in half. Cut into eight pieces.
One-half of the cucumber should be cut into 8 slices.
The radishes should be prepared ahead of time.
Place the sauce on a plate and top with the vegetables on a serving platter.

Nutritional value:
- Energy value: 186 Kcal
- Protein: 7 g
- Carbohydrates: 12 g
- Fiber: 9 g
- Sugar: 2 g
- Sodium: 4 g
- Fat: 15 g
- Of which:
- - Saturated: 5 g
- - Monounsaturated: 4 g
- - Polyunsaturated: 5 g
- - Cholesterol: 137 mg

209. GRILLED ONION-PEPPER CHEESE SANDWICH

Servings: 2
Ingredients:
1/2 medium onion
1 teaspoon olive oil
2 tablespoons whipped cream cheese
2 ounces pepper jack cheese
2 teaspoons unsalted butter
4 slices rye bread
Directions:
Place the butter to soften. Finely chop half of the onion.
Heat olive oil in a skillet over medium-high heat. Add the onion slices and stir continuously until cooked and soft. Remove the onions from the pan and set them aside.
Spread 1 tablespoon of whipped cream cheese on 2 of the bread slices, then add half of the grilled onions and cheese. Top with other slices of bread.
Spread butter on the outside of the bread slices. Grill the sandwich in a hot skillet until the bread is toasted and the cheese is melted, turning once. Cover the pan with a lid while grilling the sandwich.

Nutritional value:
- Energy value: 192 Kcal
- Protein: 19 g
- Carbohydrates: 15 g
- Fiber: 7 g
- Sugar: 3 g
- Sodium: 3 g
- Fat: 10 g
- Of which:
- - Saturated: 5 g
- - Monounsaturated: 3 g
- - Polyunsaturated: 1 g
- - Cholesterol: 127 mg

210. MICROWAVE EGG AND VEGETABLE JARS

Servings: 4
Ingredients:
4 microwave-safe pin T-size jars with lids.
8 oz. Turkey sausage
4 tablespoons shredded natural cheddar cheese
1/4 cup bell pepper
1/4 cup onion
1/4 cup broccoli
1/4 cup mushrooms
1 sparkling jalapeño bell pepper (not required)
8 large eggs
Directions:
In a small skillet cook turkey sausage until browned. Chop into crumbs as it cooks.
Prepare jars by spraying the inside with cooking spray.
Dice bell pepper, onion, broccoli and mushrooms. In a small bowl integrate the chopped vegetables. Cut the jalapeño bell pepper into slices.
Add 1/4 cup sausage, 1 tablespoon cheese, 1/4 cup diced vegetable combination and a couple or three jalapeño bell pepper slices to each jar.
Cover and store jars for up to four days in the refrigerator.
When ready to eat, beat 2 eggs, add to the jar and stir well.
Microwave for 30 seconds and stir. Repeat until eggs are set (this may also take 1-1/2 to two minutes, depending on your microwave).
Carefully remove the jar from the microwave and experiment.

Nutritional value:
- Energy value: 260Kcal
- Protein: 20g
- Carbohydrates: 3 g
- Fiber: 0g
- Sugar: 0g
- Sodium: 410mg
- Fat: 18g
- Of which:
- - Saturated: 6 g
- - Monounsaturated: 6 g
- - Polyunsaturated: 6g
- Cholesterol: 430mg

MEATS:

211. SPICY CHICKEN WINGS

Servings: 4
Ingredients:
4 onions (green)
2 tablespoons soy sauce (low sodium)
1 tablespoon of honey
1/4 cup brown sugar
2 tablespoons. Sugar (granulated)
2 tsp. all-purpose seasoning
2 teaspoons thyme (dried)
2 teaspoons chili sauce
1 teaspoon powdered ginger
1 teaspoon minced garlic
One-quarter cup apple cider vinegar
1/4 cup lime juice
Cranberry juice, 1/4 cup
Chicken wings weighing 7 pounds
Directions:
Green onions should be chopped.
Except for the chicken wings, combine all ingredients. Remove 3/4 cup of the marinade and reserve.
Place chicken wings in a large zip-top plastic bag or jar. Pour remaining marinade over wings.
Cover and marinate for 4 to 6 hours in the refrigerator.
Preheat oven to 350°F.
Bake the chicken wings for 20 minutes on a baking sheet.
Meanwhile, boil the reserved 3/4 cup marinade in a small saucepan. Reduce to 1/3 until thickened to a glaze consistency (about 10 minutes).
Remove the chicken from the oven after 20 minutes and baste the wings with the glaze.
Raise the oven temperature to 400°F and cook for another 20 minutes, or until the chicken wings are baked.

Nutritional value:
• Energy value: 186 Kcal
• Protein: 7 g
• Carbohydrates: 12 g
• Fiber: 9 g
• Sugar: 2 g
• Sodium: 4 g
• Fat: 15 g
• Of which:
• - Saturated: 5 g
• - Monounsaturated: 4 g
• - Polyunsaturated: 5 g
• - Cholesterol: 137 mg

212. WONTON QUICHE MINIS

Servings: 6
Ingredients:
1 ounce cooked lean ham
Green onions, 2 teaspoons
2 tablespoons red pepper flakes
One dozen large eggs
1 tablespoon white all-purpose flour
24 wrappers (3-1/4 "x 3") for wontons
Directions:
Preheat oven to 350°F.
Finely chop the ham. Chop green onions and red bell pepper.

In a medium bowl, mix eggs, ham, onion, bell pepper and flour until smooth. Set aside.
Lightly coat 24 miniature muffin tins with cooking oil. Gently push the center of 1 wonton wrapper into each cup, allowing the ends to stretch beyond the edges of the cup.
Fill the wonton-lined cups with the egg mixture, dividing equally among the 24 cups.
Preheat oven to 350°F and bake for 12 to 15 minutes, or until a toothpick inserted near the middle comes out clean.

Nutritional value:
• Energy value: 175 Kcal
• Protein: 13 g
• Carbohydrates: 11 g
• Fiber: 3 g
• Sugar: 2 g
• Sodium: 3 g
• Fat: 11 g
• Of which:
• - Saturated: 3 g
• - Monounsaturated: 5 g
• - Polyunsaturated: 2 g
- Cholesterol: 87 mg

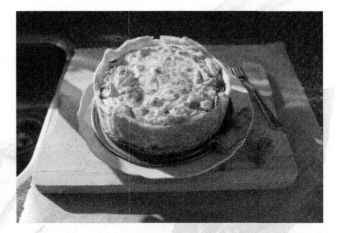

213. TURKEY BROCHETTES

Servings: 5
Ingredients:
3 pounds of turkey breasts, boneless and skinless.
6 tablespoons teriyaki sauce (low sodium)
3 teaspoons canola oil 1 1/2 teaspoons sugar
1 teaspoon powdered ginger
Nutmeg (1/2 teaspoon)
2 large onions
3 sweet bell peppers (red and green)
40 oz pineapple chunks, canned
8 oz mandarin oranges, canned
1 cup raspberry salad dressing
Grapes, 1/2 oz
Skewers or kabob sticks (24 skewers or kabob sticks).
Directions:
Cook turkey breasts for 1 hour at 350°F, or until a meat thermometer registers 180°F. Let cool.
Cut the turkey into bite-size cubes.
Combine the reduced-sodium teriyaki sauce, sugar, oil, ginger and nutmeg in a large mixing bowl.

Add the turkey cubes to the mixture. Refrigerate for 30 minutes after covering.

Onions and peppers should be cut into skewer-sized sections.

Pineapple chunks and mandarin oranges should be drained.

To make 24 kabobs, alternate turkey, onions, peppers and pineapple chunks on skewers.

Cover skewers with waxed paper in a large microwave-safe oven. 8 minutes in the microwave on skewers

Serve the skewers on a platter. Until eating, drizzle dressing over skewers and top with grapes and mandarin oranges.

Nutritional value:
- Energy value: 153 Kcal
- Protein: 7 g
- Carbohydrates: 16 g
- Fiber: 7 g
- Sugar: 5 g
- Sodium: 2 g
- Fat: 13 g
- Of which:
- - Saturated: 4 g
- - Monounsaturated: 6 g
- - Polyunsaturated: 2 g
- - Cholesterol: 115 mg

214. TEX-MEX WINGS

Servings: 5
Ingredients:
8 oz. diced green chiles in a can
1/2 cup barbecue sauce
2 teaspoons chili powder 3/4 cup honey
1/3 teaspoon cumin powder
24 drummettes of chicken wings.

Directions:
Preheat oven to 400°F.
In a large bowl, combine all Ingredients: except chicken wings.
Add chicken to coat.
Bake chicken wings for 30 to 35 minutes in a baking dish. Check to see if anything is done.
Serve wings immediately or keep warm in a covered warming dish or crockpot over low heat until ready to eat.

Nutritional value:
- Energy value: 186 Kcal
- Protein: 7 g
- Carbohydrates: 12 g
- Fiber: 9 g
- Sugar: 2 g
- Sodium: 4 g
- Fat: 15 g
- Of which:
- - Saturated: 5 g
- - Monounsaturated: 4 g
- - Polyunsaturated: 5 g
- - Cholesterol: 137 mg

215. TERIYAKI WINGS

Servings: 5
Ingredients:
24 drummettes of chicken wings
1 cup of water
1 teaspoon of cayenne pepper
2 tablespoons soy sauce (low sodium)
2-1/2 tablespoons teriyaki sauce (low sodium)
1/4 cup brown sugar
1/4 teaspoon garlic powder

One-third cup balsamic vinegar
1/2 teaspoon ginger powder.
Directions:
In a large zip-top bag, place chicken wings.
Combine all ingredients in a jar and shake to combine and coat.
Marinate overnight in the refrigerator.
Preheat oven to 400°F.
Bake chicken wings for 30 to 35 minutes in a baking dish. Check to see if anything is done.
Serve immediately or keep warm in a covered warming dish or simmer in a crockpot until ready to serve.

Nutritional value:
- Energy value: 173 Kcal
- Protein: 16 g
- Carbohydrates: 14 g
- Fiber: 7 g
- Sugar: 3 g
- Sodium: 3 g
- Fat: 10 g
- Of which:
- - Saturated: 5 g
- - Monounsaturated: 3 g
- - Polyunsaturated: 1 g
- Cholesterol: 127 mg

216. SWEET AND SOUR MEATBALLS

Servings: 5
Ingredients:
7 percent fat ground turkey, 1 lb.
One large egg
1/4 cup bread crumbs, unseasoned
2 teaspoons shallots
1 teaspoon garlic powder
One-quarter teaspoon black pepper
1/4 cup canola oil
Grape jelly, 6 oz.
1/4 cup bottled Heinz chili sauce.
Directions:
Mix ground turkey, cheese, bread crumbs, finely chopped onion, garlic powder and pepper.
To make 48 meatballs, cut the turkey mixture into 3/4-inch balls.
Heat the oil in a large skillet and cook the meatballs over medium heat. To brown evenly, turn many times. Cook until meatballs are cooked through.
In a microwave-safe dish, combine gelatin and chili sauce and heat for 1 to 2 minutes, or until gelatin is liquefied. In a warming dish or slow cooker on low heat, stir well and pour over the meatballs.

Nutritional value:
- Energy value: 192 Kcal
- Protein: 19 g
- Carbohydrates: 15 g
- Fiber: 7 g
- Sugar: 3 g
- Sodium: 3 g
- Fat: 10 g
- Of which:
- - Saturated: 5 g
- - Monounsaturated: 3 g
- - Polyunsaturated: 1 g
- - Cholesterol: 145 mg

217. SWEDISH MEATBALLS

Servings: 5
Ingredients:
1 pound onion
2 chickens, large
3 pounds of beef (ground)
1 tablespoon canola oil
1 cup raw oatmeal
1/2 cup beef broth (low sodium)
1 tablespoon dill (dried)
2 tablespoons thyme (dried)
1/4 teaspoon nutmeg
1/4 teaspoon allspice
1 teaspoon cayenne pepper
3 tablespoons butter (unsalted)
3 tablespoons all-purpose white flour
2 cups beef broth (low sodium)
1/3 cup liquid
Directions:
Preheat oven to 375°F.
Finely chop the onion. Eggs should be beaten together.
In a large bowl, combine the first 11 ingredients and stir well.
Place on a baking sheet and roll into 1" balls.
Bake for 10 to 15 minutes or until meatballs are cooked through.
In a large saucepan, melt butter to make the sauce.
Cook over medium heat, stirring constantly, until rice, reduced-sodium broth and the remaining 1 tablespoon dried thyme have thickened.
Reduce the heat to keep the meatballs warm, or place them on a covered hot plate or in a slow cooker over low heat.

Nutritional value:	
•	Energy value: 186 Kcal
•	Protein: 7 g
•	Carbohydrates: 12 g
•	Fiber: 9 g
•	Sugar: 2 g
•	Sodium: 4 g
•	Fat: 15 g
•	Of which:
•	- Saturated: 5 g
•	- Monounsaturated: 4 g
•	- Polyunsaturated: 5 g
•	- Cholesterol: 137 mg

218. MEATBALLS SOUTH OF THE BORDER

Servings: 5
Ingredients:
1/2 pound of onion
Half a cup of green peppers
2 jalapeno peppers (optional)
3 pounds of beef (ground)
5 large eggs 4 cups of cooked rice
1 tablespoon garlic powder
1 cup taco seasoning
1 liter of water
Directions:
Preheat oven to 375°F.
Chop the onion, green peppers and jalapeño peppers into small pieces. Eggs should be beaten together.
In a large bowl, combine the ground beef, onion, green bell pepper, jalapenos, cooked rice, beaten eggs and garlic powder.
Place on a baking sheet and roll into 1" balls.
Bake for 10 to 15 minutes or until meatballs are cooked through.
In a saucepan, combine taco sauce and water and bring to a boil.

Reduce heat to warm and add meatballs to taco sauce.
Serve immediately or keep warm in a covered warming dish or slow cooker on low heat.

Nutritional value:	
•	Energy value: 153 Kcal
•	Protein: 7 g
•	Carbohydrates: 16 g
•	Fiber: 7 g
•	Sugar: 5 g
•	Sodium: 2 g
•	Fat: 13 g
•	Of which:
•	- Saturated: 4 g
•	- Monounsaturated: 6 g
•	- Polyunsaturated: 2 g
•	- Cholesterol: 115 mg

219. RASPBERRY WINGS

Servings: 4
Ingredients:
2 cups raspberry preserves
3 tablespoons soy sauce (low sodium)
One-third cup of balsamic vinegar
24 drummettes of chicken wings
Directions:
Preheat oven to 400°F.
In a saucepan, heat gelatin, soy sauce and vinegar, stirring constantly until smooth.
Put the wings in a large mixing bowl. Toss the wings in the jam sauce to coat well.
In a large baking dish, coat the chicken wings with nonstick cooking spray.
Preheat oven to 350°F and bake for 30 to 35 minutes. Check to see if anything is done.
Serve wings immediately or keep warm in a covered warming dish or crockpot over low heat until ready to eat.

Nutritional value:	
•	Energy value: 175 Kcal
•	Protein: 13 g
•	Carbohydrates: 11 g
•	Fiber: 3 g
•	Sugar: 2 g
•	Sodium: 3 g
•	Fat: 11 g
•	Of which:
•	- Saturated: 3 g
•	- Monounsaturated: 5 g
•	- Polyunsaturated: 2 g
•	- Cholesterol: 87 mg

220. ITALIAN STYLE SHREDDED BEEF

Servings: 4
Ingredients:
1/2 cup onion 2 cloves garlic
2 tablespoons parsley (fresh)
Roasted veal hips, 2 pounds
1 tablespoon seasoning (Italian herbs)
1 teaspoon parsley (dried)
1 bay leaf
Half teaspoon pepper
Salt (1/4 teaspoon)
2 teaspoons extra virgin olive oil
1/2 gallon red wine
One third cup vinegar

2-3 cups water

8 rough rolls, each measuring 3-1 / 2 "in diameter and weighing 2 oz.

Directions:

Chop the onion, garlic and fresh parsley into small pieces. In a crockpot, place the roast beef. In crockpot, combine chopped onion, garlic and remaining Ingredients: (except fresh parsley and rolls); stir to combine.

Cover and cook for 8 to 10 hours on low heat or 4 to 5 hours on high heat, until tender.

Remove roast from slow cooker and set aside. Return the meat to the cooking broth to remain warm until ready to serve, shredding with two forks.

Rolls should be cut in half and served with shredded meat, fresh parsley and 1-2 tablespoons of broth. Serve as an open-faced sandwich or as an open-faced sandwich.

Nutritional value:
- Energy value: 186 Kcal
- Protein: 7 g
- Carbohydrates: 12 g
- Fiber: 9 g
- Sugar: 2 g
- Sodium: 4 g
- Fat: 15 g
- Of which:
- - Saturated: 5 g
- - Monounsaturated: 4 g
- - Polyunsaturated: 5 g
- - Cholesterol: 137 mg

221. PORK LOIN SEASONED WITH HERBS

Servings: 4

Ingredients:

2 cloves of garlic

1 teaspoon rosemary (dried)

1 teaspoon thyme (dried)

1 teaspoon basil (dried)

1 teaspoon parsley (dried)

One-fifth teaspoon black pepper

One-fourth cup Dijon mustard

1 1/2 teaspoons vegetable oil

2 pork tenderloins

Directions:

Garlic cloves should be minced. In a small bowl, combine the spices. Mix mustard and garlic together well.

Rub herb mixture generously over pork tenderloins. Refrigerate the tenderloins for at least two hours after coating.

Preheat oven to 400°F.

In a large skillet, heat the oil over medium-high heat. Cook the tenderloins in the oil until golden brown on all sides. Remove from the skillet and place in a baking dish with enough space between them so they do not touch.

Bake the tenderloins for 20 minutes or until a meat thermometer reads between 160°F (medium) and 170°F (well done) (well done).

Let the tenderloins rest for 10 to 15 minutes before slicing to allow the juices to spread evenly through the meat.

Nutritional value:
- Energy value: 175 Kcal
- Protein: 13 g
- Carbohydrates: 11 g
- Fiber: 3 g
- Sugar: 2 g
- Sodium: 3 g
- Fat: 11 g
- Of which:
- - Saturated: 3 g
- - Monounsaturated: 5 g

- - Polyunsaturated: 2 g
- - Cholesterol: 87 mg

222. KOTLET (MEAT AND POTATO EMPANADAS)

Servings: 5

Ingredients:

1 small potato

1 medium white onion

1 tablespoon of red onion

Lettuce, 3/4 cup

1 pound ground beef, lean

Single large egg

One-half teaspoon turmeric

One-fourth teaspoon garlic powder

One-fifth teaspoon black pepper

Mrs. Dash® Original Herb Seasoning Blend, 1 teaspoon

1/4 cup vegetable oil

5 pieces of 6" pita bread

One-fourth cup basil leaves.

Directions:

To minimize potassium, peel and grate potato, then soak in warm water for 2 hours. Using a clean kitchen towel, rinse, drain and squeeze out excess water.

The white onion should be grated; the red onion should be diced, and the lettuce should be shredded.

Combine the ground beef, white onion, grated potato, egg, turmeric, garlic powder, black pepper, and Mrs. Dash seasoning in a large mixing bowl until thoroughly mixed.

In a medium skillet, heat the oil.

Make 5 patties (round, about the size of your palette) and fry until browned on both sides over medium heat.

Serve each burger with lettuce, red onion and fresh basil in a pita.

Nutritional value:
- Energy value: 192 Kcal
- Protein: 19 g
- Carbohydrates: 15 g
- Fiber: 7 g
- Sugar: 3 g
- Sodium: 3 g
- Fat: 10 g
- Of which:
- - Saturated: 5 g
- - Monounsaturated: 3 g
- - Polyunsaturated: 1 g
- - Cholesterol: 127 mg

223. LISA'S AWESOME BURGERS LOW PROTEIN

Servings: 4

Ingredients:

1 pound of ground beef, lean

1 cup of finely chopped sweet onion

Single large egg

Mrs. Dash® Mesquite Grilling Mix, 3 tablespoons

6 hamburger buns

Directions:

Preheat grill as directed by the manufacturer.

Combine ground beef, onion, egg and Mrs. Dash's® seasoning in a large bowl and mix well.

Make 6 equal-sized patties with the ground beef mixture.

Grill to optimum temperature and doneness.

Serve with hamburger buns.

Nutritional value:
- Energy value: 186 Kcal
- Protein: 7 g
- Carbohydrates: 12 g
- Fiber: 9 g
- Sugar: 2 g
- Sodium: 4 g
- Fat: 15 g
- Of which:
- - Saturated: 5 g
- - Monounsaturated: 4 g
- - Polyunsaturated: 5 g
- Cholesterol: 137 mg

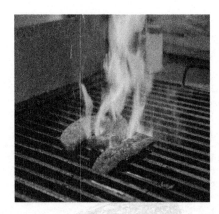

224.   MEXICAN CHORIZO

Servings: 5
Ingredients:
2 lbs. boneless pork loin, 75% lean, cubed
2 tablespoons paprika (sweet)
Chili powder (about 2 tablespoons)
1 teaspoon oregano leaves, dried
1 teaspoon cumin powder
1 teaspoon freshly ground black pepper
1/2 teaspoon cinnamon
1/2 teaspoon ground cloves
1/4 teaspoon coriander seeds
1/4 teaspoon powdered ginger
Red wine vinegar, 3 tablespoons.
Brandy (three tablespoons)
Directions:
The pork should be ground in a meat grinder with a coarse plate.
Combine the ground pork, herbs, vinegar and brandy in a large
mixing bowl. To spread the spices evenly, mix well with your hands.
Seal the chorizo in a heavy-duty plastic zip-lock bag. Refrigerate for 1
to 3 days in the very cold part of the refrigerator to allow the sausage
to cure (do not exceed 3 days). The better the flavor, the longer the
sausage will cure. The mixture can be frozen for up to 2 months for
longer storage.
Create 16 patties of the same size as the sausage. Cook the desired
portion for 10 to 15 minutes in a skillet coated with oil until browned
and cooked through.

Nutritional value:
- Energy value: 153 Kcal
- Protein: 7 g
- Carbohydrates: 16 g
- Fiber: 7 g
- Sugar: 5 g
- Sodium: 2 g
- Fat: 13 g
- Of which:
- - Saturated: 4 g
- - Monounsaturated: 6 g
- - Polyunsaturated: 2 g
- Cholesterol: 115 mg

225.   LISA'S AMAZING BURGERS

Servings: 4
Ingredients:
1 pound lean ground beef
1 cup sweet onion
One large single egg
3 tablespoons seasoning oil for hamburger Mix
4 hamburger buns
Directions:
Preheat grill to high heat.
Finely chop the onion.
Combine ground beef, onion, egg and seasoning for hamburger in a
large bowl and mix well.
Create 4 equal-sized patties with the ground beef mixture.
Grill to optimum temperature and doneness.
On hamburger buns, serve. If necessary, garnish with red onion,
thinly sliced tomato and lettuce.

Nutritional value:
- Energy value:352 Kcal
- Protein: 27g
- Carbohydrates: 27 g
- Fiber: 2g
- Sugar: 0g
- Sodium: 292mg
- Fat: 15g
- Of which:
- - Saturated: 5 g
- - Monounsaturated: 5 g
- - Polyunsaturated: 5 g
- Cholesterol: 126mg

226.   ROASTED LAMB

Servings: 4
Ingredients:
One-quarter pound butter.
1 boneless leg of lamb (about 4-1/2 pounds), well-trimmed, wrapped
and tied
1/4 cup rosemary leaves, fresh
2 cloves garlic
2 tablespoons oregano leaves, dried and crushed
1 teaspoon kosher salt
1 teaspoon freshly ground black pepper
1/4 cup freshly squeezed lemon juice
1-liter water
Directions:
Preheat oven to 325°F. Allow the butter to come to room
temperature before using.
The lamb should be washed and lightly sliced before placing in a
roasting pan.
Mince the garlic and sauté the rosemary.

In a small bowl, combine the oregano, rosemary, garlic, salt and pepper, as well as half of the softened butter or margarine.

With a sharp knife, cut slits in the leg of lamb, and push the herb and butter mixture into the slits.

Coat the lamb with the remaining herb and butter mixture.

Pour the remaining butter and lemon juice over the lamb.

Cover and bake each pound for 30 minutes.

Remove the cover after one hour, add the water to the fat in the pan and baste the meat regularly until well browned and tender.

For a crispy skin, remove the lid during the last half hour of cooking.

Nutritional value:
- Energy value: 192 Kcal
- Protein: 19 g
- Carbohydrates: 15 g
- Fiber: 7 g
- Sugar: 3 g
- Sodium: 3 g
- Fat: 10 g
- Of which:
- - Saturated: 5 g
- - Monounsaturated: 3 g
- - Polyunsaturated: 1 g
- Cholesterol: 127 mg

227. SIRLOIN TIPS GRIDDLE WITH SUMMER SQUASH AND PINEAPPLE

Servings: 5
Ingredients:
8 oz pineapple slices (canned)
2 cloves garlic
Ginger root, 2 tsp.
3 teaspoons of extra virgin olive oil
Half teaspoon salt
1 pound sirloin tips
1 medium zucchini
1 crookneck squash, medium yellow
1/2 red onion, medium
Directions:
Drain the pineapple juice and set it aside. Garlic and ginger should be minced.

In a zip-top bag, add pineapple juice, garlic, ginger, 1 teaspoon olive oil and salt. Seal the bag with the sirloin tips in the marinade.

Refrigerate at least overnight.

Preheat oven to 450°F. Foil or parchment paper with two rimmed sheet pans.

Pumpkin should be cut into 1/2-inch slices. 1 teaspoon olive oil, mixing Half of one purple onion should be cut into slices. Apply the remaining teaspoon of olive oil and stir to combine.

On one of the trays, place the pineapple rings and squash in a single layer. 5-7 minutes of roasting Switch the pineapple and squash parts after removing the pan from the oven. Add onion and roast for 4-5 minutes, or until lightly charred. Set aside, wrapped in foil to keep warm.

Remove the sirloin tips from the marinade and place them in the other pan in an even layer. Grill for 4 minutes before turning the pieces over. Cook for another 4 minutes, or until the sirloin parts are cooked through.

Serve the sirloin tips with the squash and pineapple on a platter.

Nutritional value:
- Energy value:264 Kcal
- Protein: 25g
- Carbohydrates: 14g
- Fiber: 1g
- Sugar: 0g

- Sodium: 150mg
- Fat: 12g
- Of which:
- - Saturated: 4 g
- - Monounsaturated: 4 g
- - Polyunsaturated: 4g
- Cholesterol: 74 mg

228. EASY RIBS

Servings: 5
Ingredients:
Mrs. Dash® Herb Garlic Seasoning Blend 1 tsp.
Pork ribs, 1 1/2 pounds
3 quarts of liquid
1/2 gallon of apple cider vinegar
1/4 cup barbecue sauce
Directions:
Mrs. Dash's seasoning should be evenly distributed on the top and bottom of the ribs.

Coat the top of a roasting pan with cooking spray and place the ribs in it.

Fill the bottom of the roasting pan with water and vinegar. Place the ribs on top of the pan.

Cover the ribs with aluminum foil, tucking in the corners. This allows the ribs to steam (you may need two pieces of foil to cover them completely).

Bake for 3-1/2 to 4 hours at 300°F; do not watch because it will release steam.

Brush with barbecue sauce after removing the foil. Bake for another 10 minutes in the oven.

Nutritional value:
- Energy value: 186 Kcal
- Protein: 7 g
- Carbohydrates: 12 g
- Fiber: 9 g
- Sugar: 2 g
- Sodium: 4 g
- Fat: 15 g
- Of which:
- - Saturated: 5 g
- - Monounsaturated: 4 g
- - Polyunsaturated: 5 g
- - Cholesterol: 137 mg

229. TURKEY BURGERS WITH SOUR CREAM AND ONIONS

Servings: 5
Ingredients:
1/4 medium onion
2 tablespoons chives
1 pound of turkey, 7% fat floor
1 large egg
1 tablespoon Worcestershire sauce
1 teaspoon minced garlic
1/4 teaspoon black pepper
4 tablespoons sour cream
4 split wheat hamburger buns
Directions:
Chop onion and scallions.

Combine onion, turkey, egg, Worcestershire sauce, garlic and pepper. Mix well and refrigerate for 1 hour.

Form 4 patties with the turkey mixture and refrigerate until ready to cook.

Grill the turkey patties over medium heat until cooked through, about 5 to six minutes in line with the facet. The patties are prepared while a meat thermometer registers 165°F.

Place each patty on the lower half of the bun, top with 1 tablespoon sour cream and 1/2 tablespoon chives. Place the opposite half of the bun on top and serve.

Nutritional value:
- Energy value: 350Kcal
- Protein: 29 g
- Carbohydrates:25 g
- Fiber: 2g
- Sugar: 5g
- Sodium: 326mg
- Fat: 15g
- Of which:
- - Saturated: 6 g
- - Monounsaturated: 4 g
- - Polyunsaturated: 5g
- - Cholesterol: 132mg

230. SPICY CHICKEN

Servings: 1
Ingredients:
2 tablespoons balsamic vinegar
2 tablespoons olive oil
1/4 cup green onion
1 teaspoon oregano, cleaned
1/2 teaspoon garlic powder
1/4 teaspoon black pepper
1/4 teaspoon paprika
8 oz boneless, skinless chicken breast

Starting
In a measuring cup, mix together the balsamic vinegar and olive oil. Chop the inexperienced onion and add it to the herbs and seasonings. Whisk to blend.
Cut the chicken into 2 pieces. Pour marinade over chook in a leak-proof container or plastic storage bag. Refrigerate and marinate from half an hour to 24 hours.
Remove the poultry from the marinade. Fry in a medium, nonstick or greased skillet for several minutes on each side until cooked through (using a thermometer, the internal temperature of the poultry breast should be 170° F).

Nutritional value:
- Energy value: 186 Kcal
- Protein: 7 g
- Carbohydrates: 12 g
- Fiber: 9 g
- Sugar: 2 g
- Sodium: 4 g
- Fat: 15 g
- Of which:
- - Saturated: 5 g
- - Monounsaturated: 4 g
- - Polyunsaturated: 5 g
- - Cholesterol: 137 mg

231. SLOW-ROASTED-STYLE CHICKEN

Servings: 5
Ingredients:
2 tablespoons all-purpose flour
1 large oven roasting bag
1 large onion
3 pounds whole poultry

1/4 teaspoon salt
1/4 teaspoon pepper
1 teaspoon poultry seasoning
Starting
Preheat oven to 325°F.
Shake the flour in the roasting bag.
Cut onion into slices. Place half of the onion slices inside the hollow of the chicken.
Place the bag in a roasting pan and bring the onion slices up to close. Place the bird on top of the onion.
Sprinkle the hen with salt, pepper and chicken seasoning. Close the bag according to the Directions: on the package and cut the bag in 6 places.
Bake for two hours or until the thermometer reads 165° F.
Remove from oven and let stand for 10 to fifteen minutes; open bag carefully. Remove contents to a serving dish and pour sauce from the bag into a sauce bowl.

Nutritional value:
- Energy value: 192 Kcal
- Protein: 19 g
- Carbohydrates: 15 g
- Fiber: 7 g
- Sugar: 3 g
- Sodium: 3 g
- Fat: 10 g
- Of which:
- - Saturated: 5 g
- - Monounsaturated: 3 g
- - Polyunsaturated: 1 g
- - Cholesterol: 127 mg

232. MEAT AND PEPPER PIZZA

Servings: 5
Ingredients:
1-1 / 4 teaspoons of dry yeast
1-1 / 2 cups of warm water
2 tablespoons olive oil
1 tablespoon sugar
2 cups all-purpose flour
3 ounces low sodium tomato paste
2 tablespoons Italian seasoning
1/4 teaspoon garlic powder
1/4 cup onion
1/4 cup green bell pepper
1/2 pound ground beef
1/4 teaspoon black pepper
1/4 teaspoon crushed red bell pepper
6 ounces shredded mozzarella cheese
Directions:
Preheat oven to 425°F.
Dissolve yeast in 1 cup warm water. Add 1 tablespoon olive oil, sugar and flour to make the dough. Place in a greased bowl, cover and set aside.
Combine tomato paste, 1/2 cup water, Italian seasoning, garlic powder and remaining oil in a small saucepan and simmer for 5 minutes.
Chop onion and bell pepper.
Brown meat with black pepper and crushed red bell pepper in a skillet. Drain the fat. Add the onion and green bell pepper.
Spray a pizza pan or 17 x 14-inch baking pan with nonstick cooking spray. Press dough onto pan or tray. Spread sauce, meat mixture and cheese over dough.
Bake for 20 minutes or until crust and cheese are golden brown.
Cut into 6 slices and serve.

Nutritional value:
- Energy value: 186 Kcal
- Protein: 7 g

- Carbohydrates: 12 g
- Fiber: 9 g
- Sugar: 2 g
- Sodium: 4 g
- Fat: 15 g
- Of which:
- - Saturated: 5 g
- - Monounsaturated: 4 g
- - Polyunsaturated: 5 g
- - Cholesterol: 137 mg

233. TURKEY PANINI

Servings: 1
Ingredients:
2 slices of Italian bread
2 teaspoons unsalted butter
2 slices of Sargento Ultra Thin Swiss cheese
2-1/2 ounces turkey, cooked, unsalted
2 teaspoons cranberry sauce and whole berries
Directions:
Preheat grill pan or Panini machine over medium heat.
Spread each piece of bread with 1 teaspoon of butter.
On the unbuttered side of one piece of bread, place one slice of cheese, leftover turkey slices, cranberry sauce and the remaining slice of cheese. Place the remaining slice of bread on top, butter side up.
Place sandwich in pan or Panini machine. Grill the sandwich for 5 minutes in the Panini machine or until golden brown and toasted.
If using a pan, press the sandwich down with the pan lid. Flip the sandwich after about 3 minutes or when the bottom is completely toasted. Cook the other side for about 3 minutes or until toasted.

Nutritional value:
- Energy value: 153 Kcal
- Protein: 7 g
- Carbohydrates: 16 g
- Fiber: 7 g
- Sugar: 5 g
- Sodium: 2 g
- Fat: 13 g
- Of which:
- - Saturated: 4 g
- - Monounsaturated: 6 g
- - Polyunsaturated: 2 g
- Cholesterol: 115 mg

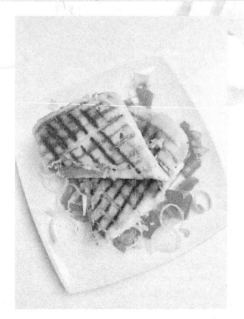

Servings: 4
Ingredients:
1/4 cup onion
1/3 cup celery
2 cups carrots
18 oz boneless, skinless turkey breast
1 teaspoon poultry seasoning
1/2 tsp chicken bouillon granules
1 cup cranberry sauce
Directions:
Dice the onion. Cut celery and carrots into slices.
Place turkey breast in a gradual cooker and sprinkle with poultry seasoning and bouillon granules.
Spoon cranberry sauce over the top; bring vegetables up.
Cover the slow cooker with a lid, turn the heat to excessive and cook dinner for 4 hours.
Remove turkey breast and cut into slices. Serve with vegetables and cranberry sauce.

Nutritional value:
- Energy value: 216Kcal
- Protein: 18g
- Carbohydrates:25 g
- Fiber: 3g
- Sugar: 4g
- Sodium: 183mg
- Fat: 1g
- Of which:
- - Saturated: 0g
- - Monounsaturated: 1 g
- - Polyunsaturated: 0g
- Cholesterol: 36 mg

235. TASTY CHICKEN EMPANADAS

Servings: 5
Ingredients:
14.5 oz of canned poultry
1 ounce of cream cheese
1 large egg
1/8 teaspoon ground sage
Half teaspoon garlic powder
Half teaspoon black pepper
1 teaspoon onion powder
1 teaspoon Italian seasoning
3/4 cup panko bread crumbs
3 tablespoons olive oil
Getting
Place the cream cheese to melt.
With a fork, mash the poultry with the juices in a medium bowl.
Add cream cheese, egg, sage, garlic powder, black pepper, onion powder, Italian seasoning and bread crumbs; mix well.
Form six patties.
In a medium skillet, heat olive oil over medium heat.
Fry patties for five to six minutes on each facet or until crisp in the open air and heated through.

Nutritional value:
- Energy value:326 Kcal
- Protein: 7g

- Carbohydrates:24 g
- Fiber: 1g
- Sugar: 1g
- Sodium: 145mg
- Fat: 22g
- Of which:
- - Saturated: 4g
- - Monounsaturated: 7 g
- - Polyunsaturated: 11g
- Cholesterol: 26mg

236. PORK CHOPS WITH PEPPER

Servings: 5
Ingredients:
1 tablespoon black peppercorns, crushed.
Pork loin chops (six)
2 teaspoons of extra virgin olive oil
Quarter cup margarine
5 cloves garlic
1 cup bell peppers (green and red)
1/2 gallon apple juice
Directions:
Peppercorns should be sprinkled and pressed on both sides of the pork chops.
In a large skillet, heat oil, margarine and garlic cloves over medium heat, stirring frequently.
Cook for 5 to 6 minutes, uncovered, with the pork chops.
Dice the bell peppers. Mix pork chops with bell peppers and apple juice.
Cover and continue cooking for another 5-6 minutes, or until pork is cooked through.

Nutritional value:
- Energy value: 186 Kcal
- Protein: 7 g
- Carbohydrates: 12 g
- Fiber: 9 g
- Sugar: 2 g
- Sodium: 4 g
- Fat: 15 g
- Of which:
- - Saturated: 5 g
- - Monounsaturated: 4 g
- - Polyunsaturated: 5 g
- - Cholesterol: 137 mg

237. PORK CHOPS WITH VEGETABLES

Servings: 4
Ingredients:
1/4 cup extra virgin olive oil
3 tablespoons basil leaves, chopped
3 tablespoons minced garlic
6 sprigs of fresh thyme
Worcestershire sauce, 1 tablespoon
Half teaspoon salt
Half teaspoon pepper
Pork chops (four)
1 pound eggplant
1 yellow squash, medium
2 carrots, medium
1 red bell pepper, medium
1/2 cup yellow onion
Directions:

In a small bowl, combine the olive oil, basil, garlic, thyme, Worcestershire sauce, salt and pepper to create the marinade.
All vegetables should be washed and cut into small pieces. Place in a large mixing bowl.
Toss vegetables in half of the marinade to coat.
Coat pork chops with remaining marinade in a tub. Refrigerate for 4 to 8 hours after covering both bowls.
Preheat oven to 400°F.
Place pork chops on one side of a rimmed skillet and vegetables on the other.
After 15 minutes of roasting, stir the vegetables. Cook for another 15 minutes, or until the pork chops reach 145 ° F.

Nutritional value:
- Energy value: 147Kcal
- Protein: 28g
- Carbohydrates:59 g
- Fiber: 8g
- Sugar: 7g
- Sodium: 1591mg
- Fat: 21g
- Of which:
- - Saturated: 7 g
- - Monounsaturated: 3 g
- - Polyunsaturated: 11g
- Cholesterol: 66 mg

238. BROCHETTES

Servings: 2
Ingredients:
1/2 cup distilled white vinegar
1/4 teaspoon black pepper
1/2 cup canola oil
1/4 teaspoon garlic powder
1/2 teaspoon oregano
1 1/2 pound beef tenderloin
2 onions, medium
2 green peppers
1 red bell pepper, chopped
Directions:
To make the marinade, mix vinegar, oil, pepper, garlic powder and oregano.
Slice beef into 1-1/2 inch thick "Cubes, to be exact. Cut the onions into quarters and cut the bell peppers into 1-1/2 inch" square-shaped pieces.
Marinate the meat and vegetables for at least 30 minutes in a sealed container.
Alternate meat and vegetables on skewers.
Grill skewers for 10 to 30 minutes over medium heat, depending on the desired degree of doneness.

Nutritional value:
- Energy value: 192 Kcal
- Protein: 19 g
- Carbohydrates: 15 g
- Fiber: 7 g
- Sugar: 3 g
- Sodium: 3 g
- Fat: 10 g
- Of which:
- - Saturated: 5 g
- - Monounsaturated: 3 g
- - Polyunsaturated: 1 g
- Cholesterol: 127 mg

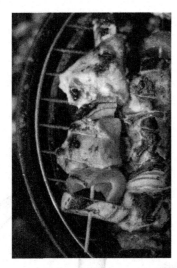

Servings: 5
Ingredients:
7 teaspoons Kikkoman® Less Sodium Teriyaki Sauce
8 ounces boneless, skinless chicken breast, uncooked
1 cup onions
1/2 cup scallions
1/2 cup lettuce
1/2 cup tomatoes
2 tablespoons olive or IL
1/3 cup low-fat mayonnaise
2 large white pita bread, 7 inches in diameter
Directions:
Place chicken in a zip-top bag. Add 5 teaspoons of teriyaki sauce and marinate in the refrigerator for 3 to 4 hours.
Dice onion; chop scallions, lettuce and tomato.
In a medium skillet, heat 1 tablespoon oil and cook chicken thoroughly until no longer pink.
Meanwhile, in a small skillet, sauté the onion in 1 tablespoon of olive oil.
While the chicken and onion are cooking, combine the mayonnaise, scallions and 2 teaspoons Kikkoman® Less Sodium teriyaki sauce. Set mixture aside.
Cut each cooked chicken breast into several strips.
Take the pita halves and coat them inside with the mayonnaise mixture. Stuff the pita with several pieces of chicken; top with the sautéed onion, lettuce and tomatoes.

Nutritional value:
- Energy value: 192 Kcal
- Protein: 19 g
- Carbohydrates: 15 g
- Fiber: 7 g
- Sugar: 3 g
- Sodium: 3 g
- Fat: 10 g
- Of which:
- - Saturated: 5 g
- - Monounsaturated: 3 g
- - Polyunsaturated: 1 g
- - Cholesterol: 127 mg

239. QUICK CHICKEN SAUTÉ

Servings: 5
Ingredients:
12 ounces of boneless, skinless poultry breast.
3 tablespoons of honey
3 tablespoons vinegar
3 tablespoons pineapple juice
1-1/2 tablespoons low-sodium soy sauce
1/2 teaspoon cornstarch
2 tablespoons canola oil
3 cups frozen mixed vegetables
3 cups warm cooked rice
Directions:
Rinse poultry; pat dry. Cut chook into 1-inch pieces; set aside.
To make the sauce, mix honey, vinegar, pineapple juice, soy sauce and cornstarch; set aside.
Pour the canola oil directly into a large skillet or wok. (Add additional oil that is important for the duration of cooking). Preheat over medium-high heat.
Stir-fry frozen vegetables for 3 minutes or until crisp-tender.
Remove vegetables from skillet.
Add chicken to the hot skillet. Stir-fry for three to four minutes or until the chicken is no longer red. Push the poultry away from the center of the skillet. Stir the sauce; move up to the center of the skillet. Cook and stir until thickened and bubbling.
Return cooked vegetables to skillet. Stir all substances to coat. Cook and stir about 1 minute more or until hot.
Serve immediately over rice.

Nutritional value:
- - Energy value: 175 Kcal
- - Protein: 13 g
- - Carbohydrates: 11 g
- - Fiber: 3 g
- - Sugar: 2 g
- - Sodium: 3 g
- - Fat: 11 g
- - Of which:
- - Saturated: 3 g
- - Monounsaturated: 5 g
- - Polyunsaturated: 2 g
- - Cholesterol: 87 mg

241. GRILLED CHICKEN PIZZA

Servings: 2
Ingredients:
1 pizza dough (see recipe from DaVita.com)
1/2 cup orange bell pepper
1/2 cup yellow bell pepper
1/4 cup red onion
1 tablespoon chives
2 tablespoons sun-dried tomato pesto
1 tablespoon olive oil
3/4 cup cooked chicken
1/3 cup shredded romano cheese
1/4 cup mozzarella cheese
Olive oil for grilling
Directions:
Dice bell peppers, onion and chives. Chop or shred the chicken.
Heat a tablespoon of olive oil and sauté the diced bell peppers and onion. Add the tomato pesto and cook for 2 minutes. Reserve for later.
Roll or stretch the pizza dough into a 10-inch circle or rectangular shape. Place on a rimless pizza pan or baking sheet (unless you are using a greased grill pizza pan). Let stand for about 5 minutes.
Grease the grill surface and preheat the grill to hot.

126

Place the pizza dough on the grill (without toppings yet) and grill for about 2 to 3 minutes. Check the bottom for browning; bubbles will form on the top. Reduce to medium-high heat if necessary to avoid burning. When light brown marks are visible on the bottom of the pizza dough, remove the dough from the grill and place the pizza dough with the grill marks facing up.

Top the pizza dough with the bell pepper, onion and pesto mixture. Top with the chicken, Romano cheese followed by the mozzarella cheese.

Return the pizza to the well-greased grill or grill pan. Grill for another 2 to 3 minutes, until the cheese, is melted and the bottom of the pizza is browned.

Remove the pizza from the grill and garnish it with chopped chives. Cut into 4 slices and serve.

Nutritional value:
- Energy value: 186 Kcal
- Protein: 7 g
- Carbohydrates: 12 g
- Fiber: 9 g
- Sugar: 2 g
- Sodium: 4 g
- Fat: 15 g
- Of which:
- - Saturated: 5 g
- - Monounsaturated: 4 g
- - Polyunsaturated: 5 g
- - Cholesterol: 137 mg

242.   CRISPY CHICKEN WRAPS

Servings: 2
Ingredients:
1 celery stalk
1 medium carrot
1/2 red bell pepper
1/4 cup low-fat mayonnaise
1/2 teaspoon onion powder
2 whole-wheat lavash or 4 whole wheat tortillas, 8-inch size
8 ounces low sodium canned chicken
Directions:
Dice celery, carrot and bell pepper.
Combine mayonnaise and onion powder in a small bowl.
Spread 2 tablespoons of the mixture on each lavash flatbread or 1 tablespoon on each tortilla.
In a separate bowl combine diced vegetables.
Place half of the vegetables and 4 ounces of chicken on one side of each flatbread. If using a tortilla, place 1/4 of the vegetables and 2 ounces of chicken on one side of each tortilla.
Roll up the flatbread and cut it in half diagonally. Secure each half with a toothpick. If using tortilla instead of lavash, secure each tortilla with a toothpick and cut each tortilla roll in half before serving.

Nutritional value:
- Energy value: 153 Kcal

- Protein: 7 g
- Carbohydrates: 16 g
- Fiber: 7 g
- Sugar: 5 g
- Sodium: 2 g
- Fat: 13 g
- Of which:
- - Saturated: 4 g
- - Monounsaturated: 6 g
- - Polyunsaturated: 2 g
- - Cholesterol: 115 mg

243.   TURKEY STUFFED GREEN PEPPERS

Servings: 4
Ingredients:
8 huge inexperienced peppers
2 pounds of floor turkey
1 cup cooked brown rice
1 tablespoon Hungarian caramel paprika
1/2 teaspoon salt
1 egg
1 medium onion, finely chopped
3 medium garlic cloves, minced
1/2 cup crushed tomatoes
1 cup low-sodium red beef broth
Starting
Preheat oven to 350°F.
Remove the stems from the peppers and smooth out the seeds and membranes inside.
Mix turkey, rice, egg, onion, garlic and seasonings together well.
Stuff the peppers with the meat combination.
Place peppers in a large roasting pan.
Pour the beaten tomatoes and broth over the peppers.
Bake for 1 hour and 15 minutes.

Nutritional value:
- Energy value: 177Kcal
- Protein: 13g
- Carbohydrates:22 g
- Fiber: 3g
- Sugar: 8g
- Sodium: 131mg
- Fat: 5g
- Of which:
- - Saturated: 3 g
- - Monounsaturated: 1 g
- - Polyunsaturated: 1g
- Cholesterol: 6 mg

DESSERTS:

244. VANILLA WAFERS WITH SWEET CREAM CHEESE SPREAD

Servings: 6
Ingredients:
8 oz whipped cream cheese
6 scoops of whey protein powder (vanilla)
Pinch of cinnamon
One-quarter teaspoon vanilla extract
A total of 72 vanilla wafer cookies
1 pound blueberries
Directions:
Combine the cream cheese, protein powder, cinnamon and vanilla extract in a stand mixer.
On each of the four vanilla wafers, spread 1 teaspoon of the cream cheese mixture.
Place 1 berry on top of each cookie.

> **Nutritional value:**
> - Energy value: 260 Kcal
> - Protein: 5 g
> - Carbohydrates: 16 g
> - Fiber: 4 g
> - Sugar: 4 g
> - Sodium: 5 g
> - Fat: 18 g
> - Of which:
> - - Saturated: 5 g
> - - Monounsaturated: 7 g
> - - Polyunsaturated: 4 g
> - - Cholesterol: 119 mg

245. SNACK MIX

Servings: 3
Ingredients:
1 cup rice cereal squares
1 cup corn cereal squares
1 cup small pretzel bagels, unsalted
3 cups of popcorn (unsalted)
One-third cup margarine, trans-fat-free
1/4 teaspoon garlic powder
1/2 teaspoon onion powder
1 tablespoon Parmigiano Reggiano
Directions:
Preheat oven to 350°F.
In a large bowl, combine cereal, pretzels and popcorn.
Melt margarine and stir in garlic and onion powder. Add the cereal mixture to the sauce to coat. Parmesan cheese should be added at this stage.
Preheat oven to 350°F and bake for 7 to 10 minutes.
Allow to cool before serving.
Keep in a hermetically sealed jar.

> **Nutritional value:**
> - Energy value: 301Kcal
> - Protein: 4g
> - Carbohydrates:38 g
> - Fiber: 2g
> - Sugar: 1g
> - Sodium:454 mg
> - Fat: 15g
> - Of which:
> - - Saturated: 2 g

> - - Monounsaturated: 3 g
> - - Polyunsaturated: 10g
> - Cholesterol: 1mg

246. SPICY CRUNCHY SNACK MIX

Servings: 3
Ingredients:
Ralston Purina Rice Chex cereal, 4 cups
2 cups of Kellogg's Crispix cereal
3 cups oyster crackers (bite-size)
1 cup pretzel bagels, unsalted
5 tablespoons unsalted margarine, trans-fat-free
1 tablespoon cayenne pepper
1/4 teaspoon cumin powder
1/4 teaspoon garlic powder
cayenne pepper, 1/8 teaspoon
Half teaspoon Worcestershire sauce
One-half teaspoon lemon juice
Directions:
Preheat oven to 250°F.
In a 10 "x 15" dish, melt margarine. Combine spices, Worcestershire sauce and lemon juice in a bowl.
Combine cereal, crackers and pretzels in a large mixing bowl. Toss to coat evenly.
Preheat oven to 350°F and bake for 45 minutes, stirring gently after 15 minutes.
To cool, spread on paper towels.
Store in an airtight jar.

> **Nutritional value:**
> - Energy value: 192 Kcal
> - Protein: 19 g
> - Carbohydrates: 15 g
> - Fiber: 7 g
> - Sugar: 3 g
> - Sodium: 3 g
> - Fat: 10 g
> - Of which:
> - - Saturated: 5 g
> - - Monounsaturated: 3 g
> - - Polyunsaturated: 1 g
> - - Cholesterol: 127 mg

247. ANISE AND ORANGE BISCOTTI

Servings: 2
Ingredients:
2 half cups of white all-purpose flour
2 teaspoons baking powder
2 teaspoons anise seeds
1 teaspoon grated orange peel
Half of 1 teaspoon sugar
2 large eggs
1/4 cup canola oil
1 teaspoon orange extract
Directions:
Preheat oven to 350°F. Line a large cookie sheet with parchment paper.
Combine the first five ingredients dry in a large bowl and stir well.

Place eggs, oil and extract in a small bowl and beat until frothy, either by hand with a whisk or with an electric mixer for about 30 seconds.
Pour the liquid aggregate into dry substances. Mix with a wooden spoon until the batter is blended. Dough may crumble.
Place dough on a lightly floured board. Form a ball and knead several times. Cut the ball in half.
Roll each half right side out into a log about 10 inches long. Flatten the top just barely.
Place dough on a cookie sheet and bake until lightly browned for about 15 to twenty minutes.
Remove from oven. Let cool for 10 minutes. Use a serrated knife and cut at about 2/3-inch intervals to make sixteen biscotti in line with half of the dough.
Place the sliced biscotti on a cookie sheet reduction side up and bake until lightly browned for about 5 minutes. Remove from oven, turn biscotti over and bake 5 minutes. Remove from oven and bake on a rack.

Nutritional value:
- Energy value: 175 Kcal
- Protein: 13 g
- Carbohydrates: 11 g
- Fiber: 3 g
- Sugar: 2 g
- Sodium: 3 g
- Fat: 11 g
- Of which:
- - Saturated: 3 g
- - Monounsaturated: 5 g
- - Polyunsaturated: 2 g
- Cholesterol: 87 mg

248. BAGEL BREAD PUDDING

Servings: 2
Ingredients:
1 medium bagel
Half cup almond milk
1/4 cup low LDL cholesterol egg alternative
1/4 cup sugar
1 teaspoon cinnamon
Starting
Preheat oven or toaster oven to 350°F. Spray a small baking dish with cooking spray.
Break bagel into small portions and place in baking dish.
Mix the almond milk, egg product, sugar and cinnamon together, then pour over the bagel pieces. Let stand for a few minutes until the bagels absorb the liquid.
Bake for half an hour or until golden brown on top. Serve warm or plain. Add whipped topping if preferred.

Nutritional value:
- Energy value: 153 Kcal
- Protein: 7 g
- Carbohydrates: 16 g
- Fiber: 7 g
- Sugar: 5 g
- Sodium: 2 g
- Fat: 13 g
- Of which:
- - Saturated: 4 g
- - Monounsaturated: 6 g
- - Polyunsaturated: 2 g
- Cholesterol: 115 mg

249. BAVARIAN APPLE PIE

Servings: 4
Ingredients:
Half cup butter
1 cup granulated sugar
3/4 teaspoon vanilla extract
1 cup white flour for all motifs
8 oz cream cheese
1 large egg
1/2 teaspoon cinnamon
4 medium apples
1/4 cup sliced almonds
Starting
Preheat oven to 450°F.
Place the cream cheese in to soften. Peel, core and slice apples.
Collectively beat butter, 1/3 cup sugar and 1/4 teaspoon vanilla.
Stir in the flour to form a dough.
Spread the dough on the bottom and sides of a nine " spring form pan.
In a medium bowl, incorporate the softened cream cheese and 1/3 cup sugar; Mix very well.
Add egg and 1/2 teaspoon vanilla; blend until blended.
Pour the mixture into a cake pan.
Combine 1/3 cup sugar and cinnamon; mix with apples until all lined.
Pour apple combination over cream cheese layer.
Sprinkle with almonds.
Bake at 450°F for 10 minutes.
Reduce temperature to 400°F and keep baking for 25 minutes. Cool.

Nutritional value:
- Energy value:287 Kcal
- Protein: 6g
- Carbohydrates:42 g
- Fiber: 4g
- Sugar: 25g
- Sodium: 508mg
- Fat: 32g
- Of which:
- - Saturated: 16 g
- -Monounsaturated: 8 g
- - Polyunsaturated: 8g
- Cholesterol: 97mg

250. FROZEN BLUEBERRY PIE

Servings: 4
Ingredients:
3/4 cup unsalted butter
1-1 / 2 cups all-purpose flour
6 tablespoons granulated sugar
3 cups whipped topping
3 ounces cream cheese
21 ounces canned blueberry pie filling.
Directions:
Preheat oven to 350°F. Set butter and cream cheese to soften.
Mix butter with flour and 2 tablespoons of sugar. Press lightly into the lowest part of a nine "x 13" x 2" glazed, ovenproof baking dish. Bake for 15 minutes or until lightly browned. Remove from oven and melt.
In a large bowl, mix cream cheese with a hand mixer until light and fluffy. Add the last of the sugar. Fold the whipped topping into the cream cheese aggregate.
Spread half of the cream cheese aggregate calmly over the cooled crust.
Frivolously spread blueberry pie filling over cream cheese combination. Spread the final cream cheese mixture calmly over the blueberries. Cover and refrigerate overnight.

Cut into 10 portions.

Nutritional value:
- Energy value: 360Kcal
- Protein: 4g
- Carbohydrates: 49g
- Fiber: 3g
- Sugar: 19 g
- Sodium: 272mg
- Fat: 17g
- Of which:
- - Saturated: 5 g
- - Monounsaturated:7 g
- - Polyunsaturated: 5 g
- Cholesterol: 0 mg

251. BLUEBERRY CREAM CONES

Servings: 3
Ingredients:
4 oz. Cream cheese
1/2 cup whipped topping
1-1 / four cup cleaned or frozen blueberries
1/4 cup blueberry jam or marmalade
6 small ice cream cones

Directions:
Soften cream cheese. Place in a bowl and beat with a mixer on high until light and fluffy.
Fold fruit and jam or preserves and whipped topping into cream cheese.
Fill cones and return to the freezer until ready to serve.

Nutritional value:
- Energy value: 150Kcal
- Protein: 4g
- Carbohydrates:24 g
- Fiber: 0g
- Sugar: 18g
- Sodium: 60mg
- Fat: 3 g
- Of which:
- - Saturated: 2g
- - Monounsaturated: 1 g
- - Polyunsaturated: 0g
- Cholesterol: 15 mg

252. CRAN-APPLE CRUMBLE

Servings: 3
Ingredients:
1 cup sparkling cranberries
3 medium apples
3/4 cup brown sugar
1 teaspoon cinnamon
Half cup whole wheat flour
Half cup granulated sugar
3 tablespoons unsalted butter

Directions:
Preheat oven to 375°F.
Cut the cranberries in half. Core, peel and coat apples.
Combine cranberries, apples, 1/4 cup packed brown sugar and cinnamon in a large bowl.
Spray a 13 "x nine" baking dish with cooking spray and pour in the cranberry mixture.
Combine flour, 1/2 cup compact brown sugar and white sugar in a medium bowl. Add butter and cut in added flour with a pastry blender or by hand. Mix well to obtain coarse crumbs.

Sprinkle topping over cranberry addition and bake for 50 minutes or until topping is golden brown.

Nutritional value:
- Energy value:117 Kcal
- Protein: 1g
- Carbohydrates: 23g
- Fiber: 3g
- Sugar: 13g
- Sodium: 4 mg
- Fat: 3g
- Of which:
- - Saturated: 2 g
- - Monounsaturated: 1 g
- - Polyunsaturated: 0 g
- Cholesterol: 7 mg

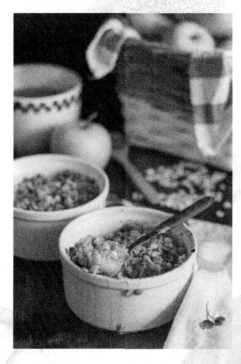

253. BAKED APPLES IN CIDER

Servings: 2
Ingredients:
4 medium baking apples
1/3 cup brown sugar
1 cup apple cider
Half teaspoon ground cinnamon
1 tablespoon unsalted butter
4 tablespoons whipping cream

Starting
Preheat oven to 350°F.
Core the apples and peel a strip from the pinnacle of each apple.
Place apples on a small baking sheet.
Combine brown sugar, cider, cinnamon and butter in a small saucepan. Bring to a boil and pour over the apples.
Bake for forty-five minutes, basting over occasion.
Serve warm. Top with whipped topping.

Nutritional value:
- Energy value: 208Kcal
- Protein: 3g
- Carbohydrates:24 g
- Fiber: 4 g
- Sugar: 2g

- Sodium: 57mg
- Fat: 5g
- Of which:
  - - Saturated:1 g
  - - Monounsaturated: 1 g
  - - Polyunsaturated: 3g
- Cholesterol: 0 mg

254.   CHEESECAKES

Servings: 4
Ingredients:
8 oz cream cheese
2 eggs
3/4 cup sugar
2 teaspoons vanilla extract
2 dozen paper cupcake liners
2 dozen vanilla wafers
1/2 cup apple pie filling
Starting
Allow cream cheese to soften for 1 hour before making tarts.
Preheat oven to 350°F.
Blend cream cheese, eggs, sugar and vanilla extract in a bowl and beat until smooth.
Place muffin tins in a muffin tin. Place a vanilla wafer in each cupcake pan.
Pour the cream cheese addition over a vanilla wafer, about 3/4 full.
Bake for 10 minutes. Remove the cakes from the oven and let them cool in the refrigerator.
Immediately before serving, top each tart with 1 half tablespoons of fruit tart filling per tart.

Nutritional value:
- Energy value: 153 Kcal
- Protein: 7 g
- Carbohydrates: 16 g
- Fiber: 7 g
- Sugar: 5 g
- Sodium: 2 g
- Fat: 13 g
- Of which:
  - - Saturated: 4 g
  - - Monounsaturated: 6 g
  - - Polyunsaturated: 2 g
  - - Cholesterol: 115 mg

255.   BLUEBERRY BLONDIES

Servings:
Ingredients:
3/4 cup butter
1-1 / 2 cups of brown sugar
2 large eggs
1 teaspoon vanilla extract
2-1 / 4 cups all-purpose flour
1-1 / 2 teaspoons baking powder
1/2 cup dried sweetened cranberries
1/3 cup white chocolate chips
8 ounces cream cheese
1-1/2 cups powdered sugar
1 teaspoon ground cinnamon
Directions:
Preheat oven to 350°F. Melt butter in a saucepan over low heat or in the microwave. Stir in the brown sugar and allow the mixture to cool to room temperature.
Place the sugar mixture in a large bowl and add the eggs and vanilla extract.

Mix the flour and baking powder and gradually add to the sugar mixture. Stir in the white chocolate and 1/3 cup blueberries.
Spray a 9 x 13-inch baking pan with cooking spray. Spread batter in pan; it will be thick Bake for 18 to 22 minutes. A toothpick inserted in the center should come out with a few crumbs. Let cool completely.
Let the cream cheese stand at room temperature for about 30 minutes. Add the cinnamon to the powdered sugar. Beat with a hand mixer for 1 minute. Gradually begin to add the powdered sugar mixture and beat until smooth.
Spread the frosting over the cooled brownies. Top with remaining blueberries. Cut into 24 pieces. Store in the refrigerator until ready to serve.

Nutritional value:
- Energy value:100 Kcal
- Protein: 3g
- Carbohydrates:13 g
- Fiber: 5g
- Sugar: 8g
- Sodium: 75mg
- Fat: 3g
- Of which:
  - - Saturated: 2 g
  - - Monounsaturated: 1 g
  - - Polyunsaturated: 0g
- Cholesterol: 15 mg

256.   CHERRY COFFEE CAKE

Servings: 5
Ingredients:
Half cup unsalted butter
2 eggs
1 cup granulated sugar
1 cup sour cream
1 teaspoon vanilla
2 cups white all-purpose flour
1 teaspoon baking powder
1 teaspoon baking soda
20 ounces cherry pie filling
Directions:
Preheat oven to 350°F. Place butter at room temperature to melt.
With a mixer, beat butter, eggs, sugar, sour cream and vanilla.
In a separate bowl, stir together flour, baking powder and baking soda.
Add the Ingredients: dry to the buttercream mixture and mix well.
Pour batter into a greased 9 "x 13" baking pan.
Spread the cherry pie filling evenly over the batter.
Bake for forty minutes until golden brown.

Nutritional value:
- Energy value: 192 Kcal
- Protein: 19 g
- Carbohydrates: 15 g
- Fiber: 7 g
- Sugar: 3 g
- Sodium: 3 g
- Fat: 10 g
- Of which:
  - - Saturated: 5 g
  - - Monounsaturated: 3 g
  - - Polyunsaturated: 1 g
- Cholesterol: 127 mg

257.   NAPOLEON BAYS

Servings: 4
Ingredients:
12 wonton wrappers
2 tablespoons granulated sugar
1 cup Reddi-Wip nonfat whipped topping
Half cup raspberries
Half cup blueberries
1 tablespoon powdered sugar
Directions:
Preheat oven to 400°F.
Spray oil spray on a baking sheet as a way to place 12 wonton wrappers.
Spread the wonton wrappers and spray them with spray oil.
Sprinkle granulated sugar on wonton wrappers.
Bake wontons for 5 minutes or until golden brown; discard on baking sheet.
Place 6 wonton wrappers on a serving platter.

Top each wrapper with 2 tablespoons whipped topping, 1 tablespoon raspberries and 1 tablespoon blueberries.
Top berries with a 2d wonton layer.
Dust the top with powdered sugar. Garnish with a dollop of whipped cream, fruit and a mint leaf, if preferred. Serve at once.

Nutritional value:
• Energy value: 175 Kcal
• Protein: 13 g
• Carbohydrates: 11 g
• Fiber: 3 g
• Sugar: 2 g
• Sodium: 3 g
• Fat: 11 g
• Of which:
• - Saturated: 3 g
• - Monounsaturated: 5 g
• - Polyunsaturated: 2 g
• - Cholesterol: 87 mg

Bases:

258. SHRIMP CREAM WITH CRACKERS

Servings: 2
Ingredients:
1/4 cup cream cheese (light)
2 1/2 oz shelled fried shrimp, shells removed
1 tablespoon tomato sauce (no salt added)
Tabasco hot sauce, 1/4 tsp.
1 teaspoon Worcester sauce
Half teaspoon Mrs. Dash is a spice seasoning blend made by Mrs. Dash.
Miniature matzah crackers (24).
1 teaspoon parsley
Directions:
Let the cream cheese melt in the refrigerator.
In a bowl, chop shrimp and add to cream cheese.
Combine the tomato sauce, Tabasco sauce, Worcestershire sauce and herb seasoning in a large mixing bowl.
On each cracker, spread 1 teaspoon of the spread. Garnish with chopped parsley.

Nutritional value:	
•	Energy value: 192 Kcal
•	Protein: 19 g
•	Carbohydrates: 15 g
•	Fiber: 7 g
•	Sugar: 3 g
•	Sodium: 3 g
•	Fat: 10 g
•	Of which:
•	- Saturated: 5 g
•	- Monounsaturated: 3 g
•	- Polyunsaturated: 1 g
•	- Cholesterol: 127 mg

259. VEGETABLE LAYER

Servings: 4
Ingredients:
7 slices of sourdough bread, 1/2 "thick.
1 tablespoon unsalted margarine
1 cup onion
1 cup raw mushrooms
1 cup bell peppers
15 fresh spinach leaves
7 large eggs
1/4 cup tarragon vinegar
1-3/4 cups half and half cream
1 teaspoon Worcestershire sauce
1 teaspoon warm Tabasco sauce
1/2 teaspoon black pepper
1 ounce shredded sharp cheddar cheese
Directions:
Cut bread into cubes. Place on a baking sheet and bake at 225°F for 15 minutes. Turn cubes over and continue baking for 15 minutes or until dry and crisp.
Dice the onion, mushrooms and bell peppers.
Melt the margarine in a small skillet and sauté the onion, mushrooms and crimson peppers.

Grease a 9" rectangular baking dish with nonstick cooking spray. Place half of the bread cubes in a single layer in the dish and sprinkle with half of the vegetable combination. Place spinach leaves on top. Form a second layer with the best bread and greens on top.
Whisk collectively the eggs, vinegar, half and half cream, Worcestershire sauce, warm sauce and black pepper. Pour evenly over the bread.
Cover surface with plastic wrap and refrigerate for at least 1 hour or overnight.
Let the strata stand up to room temperature for 20 minutes.
Preheat oven to 325°F. Remove plastic wrap and bake for 50 minutes.
Remove from oven and sprinkle cheddar cheese over the pinnacle. Bake for 10 minutes more or until a knife inserted near the center comes out clean.
Cut into nine portions and serve hot.

Nutritional value:	
•	Energy value:156 Kcal
•	Protein: 6g
•	Carbohydrates:19 g
•	Fiber: 7g
•	Sugar: 3 g
•	Sodium: 280mg
•	Fat: 8g
•	Of which:
•	- Saturated: 5 g
•	- Monounsaturated: 2 g
•	- Polyunsaturated: 1 g

- Cholesterol: 0mg

260. SEAFOOD DIP

Servings: 5
Ingredients:
Cream cheese, 8 oz
8 oz frozen cooked shrimp (any size)
4 oz of crab meat
Added 1 cup Hunt's® unsalted tomato sauce
1 1/2 teaspoons horseradish, prepared
1/4 cup lemon juice
1 tablespoon Worcestershire sauce (low sodium)
Tabasco® hot sauce, 1/2 tsp.
30 low sodium saltine crackers.
Directions:
To soften cream cheese, remove from refrigerator. Microwave softening is not recommended.
Thaw shrimp according to Directions: on the product. Break shrimp into small pieces after removing shells and visible veins.
Prepare imitation crab meat by cutting it into small pieces.
Refrigerate the shrimp and crab meat after mixing.
To make a low-sodium cocktail sauce, mix ketchup, horseradish, lemon juice and Worcestershire sauce in a small cup.
Stir softened cream cheese until smooth in a medium cup.
Add cocktail sauce to cream cheese in a slow, steady stream. Stir everything together thoroughly.
Mix the cream cheese with a pinch of Tabasco® sauce. Stir everything together thoroughly. Take a bite of the cream cheese mixture. As needed, add more Tabasco® sauce.
Mix cream cheese with shrimp and crab meat. Stir everything together thoroughly. Take a bite of the cream cheese mixture. As needed, add more Tabasco® sauce.
Refrigerate overnight after covering.

Serve with low sodium crackers as a garnish.

Nutritional value:
- Energy value: 110Kcal
- Protein: 5g
- Carbohydrates:4 g
- Fiber: 0g
- Sugar: 1 g
- Sodium: 291mg
- Fat: 8g
- Of which:
- - Saturated: 5 g
- - Monounsaturated: 2 g
- - Polyunsaturated: 1g
- Cholesterol: 22 mg

261. SPICY CORNBREAD

Servings: 4
Ingredients:
1 cup white all-purpose flour
1 cup of undeniable cornflour
1 tablespoon of sugar
2 teaspoons baking powder
1 teaspoon chili powder
1/4 teaspoon black pepper
1 cup rice milk, not enriched
1 egg
1 egg white
2 tablespoons canola oil
1/2 cup scallions, finely chopped
1/4 cup carrots, Finely Grated
1 clove garlic, minced
Directions:
Preheat oven to 400°F.
In a large bun, integrate flour, cornmeal, sugar, baking powder, chili powder and pepper. Stir to mix.
Add rice milk, egg, egg white and oil to Ingredients: dry and stir until moistened d.
Gently stir scallions, carrots and garlic into a cornbread combination.
Pour batter into an eight-inch square baking pan that has been lined with nonstick cooking spray.
Bake for 25 to 30 minutes, until the pinnacle, begins to evolve to show a golden brown color. Cut into 8 2" x 4" pieces.

Nutritional value:
- Energy value:160 Kcal
- Protein: 3g
- Carbohydrates:25 g
- Fiber: 1g
- Sugar: 10g
- Sodium: 320mg
- Fat: 6g
- Of which:
- - Saturated: 3 g
- - Monounsaturated: 2 g
- - Polyunsaturated: 1 g
- Cholesterol: 15 mg

262. PIONEER PUMPKIN BREAD

Servings: 5
Ingredients:
3 halves of cups of white flour for all motifs
3 cups of sugar
3 teaspoons of baking soda

1 teaspoon salt
1 teaspoon cinnamon on the ground
1 teaspoon nutmeg
1 cup oil
2/3 cup water
4 eggs
15 ounce can of pumpkin
Directions:
Preheat oven to 350°F.
Mix Ingredients: dry in a large bowl. Add oil, water, eggs and pumpkin. Stir until well combined. Add nuts, if preferred.
Pour batter into loaf pans, lightly sprayed with nonstick cooking spray.
To make 3 regular-sized loaves, bake for 1 hour or until a toothpick inserted in the middle comes out clean. To make 6 small loaves, bake for 45 minutes.
Cool loaves on a rack for 10 minutes in pans; then invert, remove from pans and turn appropriate aspect up and keep cooling. Wrap in foil when completely cool.

Nutritional value:
- Energy value: 192 Kcal
- Protein: 19 g
- Carbohydrates: 15 g
- Fiber: 7 g
- Sugar: 3 g
- Sodium: 3 g
- Fat: 10 g
- Of which:
- - Saturated: 5 g
- - Monounsaturated: 3 g
- - Polyunsaturated: 1 g
- Cholesterol: 127 mg

263. ZUCCHINI BREAD

Servings: 5
Ingredients:
3 cups of white all-purpose flour
3/4 cups sugar or Splenda granulated sweetener
1 1/2 teaspoons pumpkin pie spice
1-half teaspoons of baking soda
1 teaspoon salt
4 eggs
2 cups shredded zucchini
3/4 cup honey
1/3 cup oil
1/3 cup unsweetened applesauce
2 tablespoons lemon juice
1 teaspoon vanilla extract
Directions:
Preheat oven to 325°F.
Grease 8 " x 4 " loaf pan halves.
In a large bowl, whisk together flour, sugar, pumpkin pie spice, baking soda and salt.
In a medium bowl, beat the eggs barely. Add the zucchini, honey, oil, applesauce, lemon juice and vanilla.
Stir liquid combination into flour combination until flour is moistened. Spread evenly into loaf pans.
Bake for 1 hour or until the toothpick comes out easily.
Cool in pan on wire racks for 10 minutes, then remove from pans.
Cut each loaf into 12 slices.

Nutritional value:
- Energy value: 220Kcal
- Protein: 4g
- Carbohydrates:32 g
- Fiber: 1g
- Sugar: 17g
- Sodium: 260mg

- Fat: 9g
- Of which:
- - Saturated: 5 g
- - Monounsaturated: 2 g
- - Polyunsaturated: 2g
- Cholesterol: 30 mg

264. PUMPKIN BREAD

Servings: 4
Ingredients:
2 cups sugar
2 cups of canned pumpkin
2/3 cups of water
4 large eggs
1/2 cup cooking oil
1/2 teaspoon baking powder
1 teaspoon cinnamon
1 teaspoon ginger
1 teaspoon salt
2 teaspoons of baking soda
Three half cups of white flour for all causes
Directions:
Preheat oven to 350° F.
In a large bowl, whisk together the sugar, pumpkin, water, eggs and oil.
Add the baking powder, cinnamon, ginger, salt, baking soda and flour. Stir until clean.
Pour batter into 3 loaf pans and bake for 45 minutes or until a toothpick inserted comes out easily.
Cool loaves inside the pans for 10 minutes, then turn out and cool on wire racks. Cut each loaf into 10 slices while preparing to serve.

Nutritional value:
- Energy value: 175 Kcal
- Protein: 13 g
- Carbohydrates: 11 g
- Fiber: 3 g
- Sugar: 2 g
- Sodium: 3 g
- Fat: 11 g
- Of which:
- - Saturated: 3 g
- - Monounsaturated: 5 g
- - Polyunsaturated: 2 g
- - Cholesterol: 87 mg

265. STRAWBERRY BREAD

Servings: 5
Ingredients:
2 cup halves of carbonated strawberries or 14 ounces of frozen strawberries, no sugar added
3 cups white flour for all purposes
2 cups granulated sugar
1 teaspoon of baking soda
1/4 teaspoon cinnamon powder
3/4 teaspoon salt
Four large eggs
1 cup canola oil
Directions:
Preheat oven to 350°F.
Finely chop the strawberries.
In a medium bowl, whisk the eggs. Add canola oil and strawberries and stir well.
Mix Ingredients: dry in a separate large bowl.
Make a nice inside center of the dry ingredients and pour into the egg mixture.

Use a large spoon and mix until well combined; do not overmix now. Pour batter into two ungreased 9 "x 5" loaf pans. Bake for 50 to 60 minutes.
Let cool for 15 minutes, then use a knife to loosen the perimeters of the loaf from the loaf pans and loosen them slightly. Finish cooling on a wire rack.
Serve or wrap the bread in plastic wrap or aluminum foil to keep it clean. Bread can be refrigerated or frozen.

Nutritional value:
- Energy value: 173Kcal
- Protein: 3 g
- Carbohydrates: 30g
- Fiber: 1 g
- Sugar: 19g
- Sodium: 240mg
- Fat: 5g
- Of which:
- - Saturated: 3 g
- - Monounsaturated: 1 g
- - Polyunsaturated: 1 g
- Cholesterol: 24mg

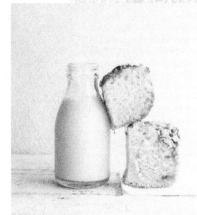

266. FRESH HERB CRANBERRY FILLING

Servings: 4
Ingredients:
1/2 cup onion
1/2 cup celery
1/2 tablespoon fresh parsley
1/2 tablespoon fresh sage
1/2 tablespoon fresh rosemary
1/2 tablespoon fresh thyme
8 slices bread
1/4 cup unsalted butter
1/2 teaspoon black pepper
2 teaspoons poultry seasoning
1/2 cup sweetened dried cranberries
1/2 cup low-cholesterol liquid egg substitute
1/4 cup chicken or turkey broth
Directions:
Chop onion and celery. Chop fresh herbs. Cut bread into 1/2 inch cubes.
Melt butter in a nonstick skillet. Sauté onion and celery until tender. Remove from heat.
Stir in cubed bread, pepper, poultry seasoning, fresh herbs and cranberries.
Mix egg product and broth together. Pour into the bread mixture and mix lightly.

Place stuffing in the turkey body cavity and neck cavity to cook, or bake stuffing separately in a baking dish sprayed with nonstick cooking spray at 350° F for 45 minutes.

Nutritional value:
- Energy value: 192 Kcal
- Protein: 19 g
- Carbohydrates: 15 g
- Fiber: 7 g
- Sugar: 3 g
- Sodium: 3 g
- Fat: 10 g
- Of which:
- - Saturated: 5 g
- - Monounsaturated: 3 g
- - Polyunsaturated: 1 g
- - Cholesterol: 127 mg

267. DELICIOUS YOGURT AND FRUIT DIP

Servings: 4
Ingredients:
Light cream cheese, 4 oz.
6 ounces vanilla-flavored low-fat Greek yogurt
Strawberry fruit spread, 1/4 cup Polaner® All Fruit with Fiber
Pinch of cinnamon
Splenda® zero-calorie sweetener, 6 packets
Directions:
In a medium bowl, blend Ingredients: with a hand mixer until smooth.
Place in refrigerator until ready to eat.

Nutritional value:
- Energy value: 153 Kcal
- Protein: 7 g
- Carbohydrates: 16 g
- Fiber: 7 g
- Sugar: 5 g
- Sodium: 2 g
- Fat: 13 g
- Of which:
- - Saturated: 4 g
- - Monounsaturated: 6 g
- - Polyunsaturated: 2 g
- Cholesterol: 115 mg

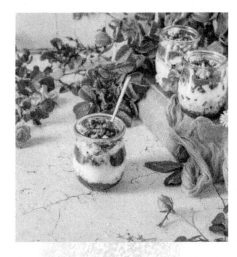

268. PIZZA DOUGH

Servings: 3
Ingredients:
2 cups warm water
1 package active dry yeast (0.25 ounces)
1 tablespoon plus 1 pinch of sugar
5 cups flour for all purposes
1/2 teaspoon salt
2 tablespoons olive oil
Directions:
In a small bowl combine the water, yeast and a pinch of sugar; stir lightly. Let the combination sit for a couple of minutes to activate (it will bubble).
In a blender bowl combine flour, remaining 1 tablespoon sugar, salt and 2 tablespoons olive oil; stir well. Add yeast addition to the flour mixture; stir well.
Knead the dough. Use a mixer with a dough attachment or knead on a floured floor until clean and easily rolled out. Grease the bottom and sides of a bowl and place the dough inside. Loosen Ly cowl the bowl with a paper towel or kitchen towel.
Place the bowl covered with a blanket on the stove and let the dough push up until it doubles in length for 1 half to 2 hours. Punch down the dough and divide it into 5 equal parts.
Stretch each piece of pizza dough into a ten-inch circle or square shape to gather them together for pizza toppings.

Nutritional value:
- Energy value:72 Kcal
- Protein: 2 g
- Carbohydrates:10 g
- Fiber: 1 g
- Sugar: 1g
- Sodium: 102mg
- Fat: 1g
- Of which:
- - Saturated: 0 g
- - Monounsaturated: 0 g
- - Polyunsaturated: 1g
- Cholesterol: 0 mg

DRINKS:

269. PINEAPPLE PONCHET

Servings: 4
Ingredients:
1 gallon of pineapple juice
2 liters of ginger ale or lemon-lime soda
8 oz crushed pineapple in a can
Pineapple slices for garnish 4 cups of ice cubes (optional)
Directions:
In a large punch bowl, combine all ingredients.
In a punch bowl or other clear bottle, serve.
If necessary, garnish with pineapple slices on the rim of the bottle.

> **Nutritional value:**
> - Energy value: 192 Kcal
> - Protein: 19 g
> - Carbohydrates: 15 g
> - Fiber: 7 g
> - Sugar: 3 g
> - Sodium: 3 g
> - Fat: 10 g
> - Of which:
> - - Saturated: 5 g
> - - Monounsaturated: 3 g
> - - Polyunsaturated: 1 g
> - - Cholesterol: 127 mg

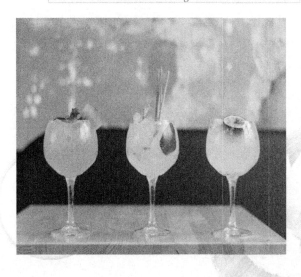

270. POWER PUNCH

Servings: 4
Ingredients:
4 ounces chilled cranberry tangerine juice
1 heaping scoop (6.6 g) ProCel® whey protein powder
Sugar (two teaspoons)
1/2 cup ice cubes
Directions:
In a blender, combine cranberry and tangerine juice, whey powder, sweetener and ice until pink and frothy.
Pour immediately into a glass and serve.

> **Nutritional value:**
> - Energy value: 500Kcal
> - Protein: 10g
> - Carbohydrates:113 g

> - Fiber: 4g
> - Sugar: 0g
> - Sodium: 91mg
> - Fat: 2g
> - Of which:
> - - Saturated: 2g
> - - Monounsaturated: 0 g
> - - Polyunsaturated: 0 g
> - Cholesterol: 2 mg

271. PURPLE PONCH

Servings: 4
Ingredients:
2 quarts (64 oz.) ginger ale.
4 six-ounce cans of frozen grape juice concentrate, thawed
2 pints of lime sherbet
Raspberry sorbet, 2 pints.
Directions:
In a large punch bowl, combine the ginger ale and grape juice concentrate.
Mix the sherbet into the punch and stir to combine.

> **Nutritional value:**
> - Energy value: 175 Kcal
> - Protein: 13 g
> - Carbohydrates: 11 g
> - Fiber: 3 g
> - Sugar: 2 g
> - Sodium: 3 g
> - Fat: 11 g
> - Of which:
> - - Saturated: 3 g
> - - Monounsaturated: 5 g
> - - Polyunsaturated: 2 g
> - - Cholesterol: 87 mg

272. SPICED EGGNOG

Servings: 2
Ingredients:
2 cups half-and-half cream
One-third cup of low-cholesterol egg product
2 teaspoons rum extract 1/4 cup sugar
1/2 tsp. pumpkin pie spice
One-fifth teaspoon nutmeg
Whipping cream, 6 tablespoons.
Directions:
In a cold blender, combine the half-and-half, cream, egg product, sugar, rum extract and pumpkin pie spice and blend for 1 to 2 minutes.
Pour mixture into 6 tiny glasses. Add a tablespoon of whipped topping and a pinch of nutmeg to each serving.

> **Nutritional value:**
> - Energy value:264 Kcal
> - Protein: 9g
> - Carbohydrates: 15g
> - Fiber: 0g
> - Sugar: 15 g
> - Sodium:103 mg

- Fat: 8g
- Of which:
- - Saturated: 5 g
- - Monounsaturated: 1 g
- - Polyunsaturated: 2g
- Cholesterol: 112 mg

273. DREAMSICLE STRAWBERRY DELIGHT

Servings: 4
Ingredients:
2 quarts almond milk
3 scoops Syntrax Nectar Vanilla Bean Torte Whey Protein Isolate Powder
Torani sugar-free vanilla syrup, 1/4 cup
Strawberry extract (two teaspoons)
1/2 cup strawberry soda (sugar-free).
Directions:
In a blender, combine almond milk and protein powder. Blend well. Stir in strawberry extract.
Pour mixture into four cups, then slowly apply two scoops of strawberry soda to each cup. Have fun

Nutritional value:
- Energy value: 153 Kcal
- Protein: 7 g
- Carbohydrates: 16 g
- Fiber: 7 g
- Sugar: 5 g
- Sodium: 2 g
- Fat: 13 g
- Of which:
- - Saturated: 4 g
- - Monounsaturated: 6 g
- - Polyunsaturated: 2 g
- Cholesterol: 115 mg

274. STRAWBERRY AND APPLE JUICE BLEND

Servings: 4
Ingredients:
1 pound of strawberries
1 medium apple
6 mint leaves
A quarter of a lemon
Green tea, 4 oz.
Directions:
In a juicer, combine strawberries, apple, mint and lemon to extract the juice. Pour in the green tea.
To make two servings, pour the mixture into two small glasses. Drink immediately or chill in the refrigerator.

Nutritional value:
- Energy value: 227 Kcal
- Protein: 5 g
- Carbohydrates: 7 g
- Fiber: 5 g
- Sugar: 3 g
- Sodium: 2 g
- Fat: 9 g
- Of which:
- - Saturated: 7 g
- - Monounsaturated: 1 g
- - Polyunsaturated: 1 g

- - Cholesterol: 100 mg

275. STRAWBERRY HIGH PROTEIN SOFT FRUIT

Servings: 2
Ingredients:
New strawberries, 3/4 cup
Pasteurized liquid egg whites, 1/2 cup
1/2 cup ice
Sugar, 1 tablespoon
Directions:
Blend strawberries until completely smooth in a blender.
Add the rest of the ingredients until smooth.

Nutritional value:
- Energy value: 192 Kcal
- Protein: 19 g
- Carbohydrates: 15 g
- Fiber: 7 g
- Sugar: 3 g
- Sodium: 3 g
- Fat: 10 g
- Of which:
- - Saturated: 5 g
- - Monounsaturated: 3 g
- - Polyunsaturated: 1 g
- - Cholesterol: 127 mg

276. SUPER FRUIT SMOOTHIE

Servings: 4
Ingredients:
8 fluid ounces of Nepro refrigerated vanilla Nepro with Stead carb.
2 scoops whey protein isolate
1 cup peaches or mixed berries, frozen
Optional: 1/2 cup crushed ice
Directions:
Blend frozen fruit in a blender.
Combine chilled Nepro, whey protein and crushed ice in a blender (if desired).
Blend until completely smooth.
Pour into a bottle and top with a straw to serve.

Nutritional value:
- Energy value: 153 Kcal
- Protein: 7 g
- Carbohydrates: 16 g
- Fiber: 7 g
- Sugar: 5 g
- Sodium: 2 g
- Fat: 13 g
- Of which:
- - Saturated: 4 g
- - Monounsaturated: 6 g
- - Polyunsaturated: 2 g
- - Cholesterol: 115 mg

277. VANILLA MILK ALTERNATIVE

Servings: 3
Ingredients:
8 ounces heavy whipping cream 6 1/2 cups cold water.
6 scoops whey protein powder 100 percent EAS, vanilla
Directions:

Blend 1/4 to 1/2 of the recipe in a blender for 20 seconds at a time (depending on the size of your blender) to fully incorporate the protein powder.
Enjoy the cold version!

Nutritional value:
- Energy value: 175 Kcal
- Protein: 13 g
- Carbohydrates: 11 g
- Fiber: 3 g
- Sugar: 2 g
- Sodium: 3 g
- Fat: 11 g
- Of which:
- - Saturated: 3 g
- - Monounsaturated: 5 g
- - Polyunsaturated: 2 g
- - Cholesterol: 87 mg

278. VANILLA ROOT BEER DELIGHT

Servings: 4
Ingredients:
2 quarts almond milk
Vanilla Bean, 3 scoops Syntrax Nectar Whey Protein Isolate Powder Cake flavor
Torani sugar-free vanilla syrup, 1/4 cup
2 teaspoons root beer flavoring
1/2 cup root beer soda (diet).
Directions:
In a blender, combine almond milk and protein powder. Blend well. Stir in the root beer extract.
Pour mixture into four cups and slowly add 2 teaspoons of root beer soda. have fun!

Nutritional value:
- Energy value:129 Kcal
- Protein: 18g
- Carbohydrates:12 g
- Fiber: 0 g
- Sugar: 0g
- Sodium: 145mg
- Fat: 1g
- Of which:
- - Saturated: 0g
- - Monounsaturated: 0 g
- - Polyunsaturated: 1 g
- Cholesterol: 0mg

279. WATERMELON AGUA FRESCA

Servings: 2
Ingredients:
2 cups seedless watermelon
1 cup water
1 tablespoon sugar
2 sprigs of mint leaves
1 lime (for garnish)
Directions:
Cut the lime into thin slices. Watermelon should be cut into large chunks and measured into 2 cups.
Blend the watermelon and 2 lime slices in a blender until smooth. Strain the mixture through a strainer into 4 cups. Serve garnished with mint leaves and lime slices.

Nutritional value:
- Energy value:92 Kcal
- Protein:2 g
- Carbohydrates: 21g
- Fiber: 2g
- Sugar: 0g
- Sodium: 8mg
- Fat: 0 g
- Of which:
- - Saturated: 0 g
- - Monounsaturated: 0 g
- - Polyunsaturated: 0g
- Cholesterol: 0 mg

280. VANILLA SMOOTHIE

Servings: 4
Ingredients:
1 cup sugar (or sugar substitute).
Vanilla extract (1/4 teaspoon)
8 oz liquid egg white (pasteurized)
Whipped topping, 3 tablespoons
Directions:
Both Ingredients: must be combined.
Mix until a perfectly melted whipped topping is achieved.

Nutritional value:
- Energy value: 227 Kcal
- Protein: 5 g
- Carbohydrates: 7 g
- Fiber: 5 g
- Sugar: 3 g
- Sodium: 2 g
- Fat: 9 g
- Of which:
- - Saturated: 7 g
- - Monounsaturated: 1 g
- - Polyunsaturated: 1 g
- Cholesterol: 100 mg

FREE DOWNLOAD
Plant Based Keto

Dear reader, if you're reading this sentence, you probably haven't carefully read the description of this book on the Amazon page, where the link to buy the COLOR version is clearly indicated at the end.

But don't worry, I have a surprise for you:

SCAN THE QR CODE TO DOWNLOAD AND ENJOY THE COLOR VERSION!

Plan Renal

WEEK N°1

Monday	Breakfast: • 3 Zucchini Muffins Snack: • 1 Tomato jar appetizer Lunch: • A couple of eggs stuffed with shrimp • 3½ oz of raw vegetables and salsa • A power punch Snack: • 1¾ oz of popcorn with sugar and spices. Dinner: • Grilled onion and pepper cheese sandwich.
Tuesday	Breakfast: • 2 Super simple baked pancakes Snack: • 1 sweet popcorn ball Lunch: • A couple of individual frittatas • Microwavable egg and vegetable jars • 1 Cup of Dreamsicle Strawberry Delight Snack: • One vanilla wafer with sweet cream cheese spread Dinner: • 2 Kotlet (meat and potato patties).
Wednesday	Breakfast: • 2 Maple pancakes Snack: • Sweet and spicy tortilla chips Lunch: • One pita pocket roll • 9 oz of shredded beef Italian style • 1 glass of strawberry-apple juice blend Snack: • One cup of snack mix Dinner: • 2 Stuffed French toast
Thursday	Breakfast: • 1 Cup of blueberries in snow. Snack: • 1 Anise and orange biscotti. Lunch: • 2 Omelet wraps • A couple of spicy chicken wings • One vanilla root beer delight Snack: • Bagel bread pudding Dinner: • One of Lisa's mind-blowing burgers.
Friday	Breakfast: • 3 apple bars Snack:

	• A Bavarian apple pie
	Lunch:
	    • One samosa
	    • A couple of Tex-Mex wings
	    • A glass of Watermelon Agua Fresca
	Snack:
	    • A super fruit smoothie
	Dinner:
	    • A slab of sirloin tips with summer squash and pineapple.

Saturday	Breakfast:
	    • 2 blueberry and peach crisp.
	Snack:
	    • One frozen blueberry cobbler
	Lunch:
	    • Fettuccini Alfredo
	Snack:
	    • A sweet ball of popcorn
	Dinner:
	    • One grilled chicken pizza

Sunday	Breakfast:
	    • 1 Cup of rice pudding
	Snack:
	    • 3½ oz of blueberry cream cones.
	Lunch:
	    • A couple of tortilla rolls
	    • 3 Skewers of turkey
	Snack:
	    • One cran-apple crumble
	Dinner:
	A turkey burger with sour cream and onions.

WEEK N°2

Monday	Breakfast: • 2 soft pretzels Snack: • 1 baked apple in cider Lunch: • Teriyaki wings • Tortilla rolls. Snack: • 1 Cheesecake Dinner: • A couple of empanadas with meat.
Tuesday	Breakfast: • One anise and orange biscotti. • Two apple bars Snack: • One blueberry blondie Lunch: • One wonton Quiche Minis Snack: • 1¾ oz of popcorn with sugar and spices. Dinner: • One meat and pepper pizza
Wednesday	Breakfast: • Cream of shrimp soup with crackers Snack: • Cherry pie Coffee Lunch: • 3 Sweet and sour meatballs • 2 slices of spicy cornbread Snack: • A cup of Napoleon berries Dinner: • One Turkey panini
Thursday	Breakfast: • Two slices of pioneer pumpkin bread with cream cheese. Snack: • One anise and orange biscotti. Lunch: • 1 Pork tenderloin seasoned with herbs. Snack: • A super fruit smoothie Dinner: • One turkey breast in the slow cooker with carrots and cranberry sauce.
Friday	Breakfast: • Two slices of zucchini bread with blueberry stuffing. Snack: • 1 Zucchini muffin Lunch: • Swedish meatballs Snack: • A strawberry drink high protein fruit Suave. Dinner: • 2 Kotlet (meat and potato patties).
Saturday	Breakfast: • A delicious yogurt and fruit dip. Snack:

	• A vanilla milkshake
	Lunch:
	• 3 Meatballs south of the border.
	• Vegetables
	Snack:
	• 1¾ oz of popcorn
	Dinner:
	• 2 Tasty chicken empanadas
Sunday	Breakfast:
	• 3-4 Zucchini muffins
	Snack:

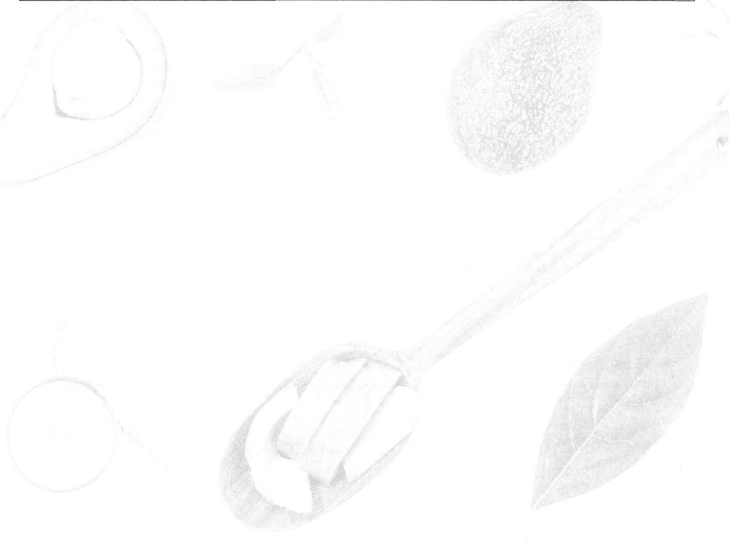

Printed in Great Britain
by Amazon